Putting Risk in Perspective

Putting Risk in Perspective

Black Teenage Lives in the Era of AIDS

Renée T. White

ROWMAN & LITTLEFIELD PUBLISHERS, INC.
Lanham • Boulder • New York • Oxford

ROWMAN & LITTLEFIELD PUBLISHERS, INC.

Published in the United States of America
by Rowman & Littlefield Publishers, Inc.
4720 Boston Way, Lanham, Maryland 20706

12 Hid's Copse Road
Cumnor Hill, Oxford OX2 9JJ, England

British Library Cataloguing in Publication Information Available

Library of Congress Cataloging-in-Publication Data

White, Renée T.
    Putting risk in perspective : Black teenage lives in the era of
AIDS / Renée T. White.
        p.   cm.
    Includes bibliographical references and index.
    ISBN 0-8476-8586-1 (cloth : alk. paper).—ISBN 0-8476-8587-X
(pbk. : alk. paper)
    1. Afro-American teenage girls—Sexual behavior. 2. Afro-American
teenage girls—Social conditions. 3. Afro-American teenage girls—
Health risk assessment. 4. Afro-American testing girls—
Connecticut—New Haven—Case studies. 5. AIDS (Disease)—Social
aspects—United States. 6. AIDS (Disease) in adolescence—United
States. 7. Safe sex in AIDS prevention—United States. 8. Health
behavior in adolescence—United States. I. Title.
HQ27.5.W48   1999
306.7'0835'2—dc21   98-28145
                                                              CIP

Printed in the United States of America

∞ ™ The paper used in this publication meets the minimum requirements of
American National Standard for Information Sciences—Permanence of Paper
for Printed Library Materials, ANSI Z39.48–1984.

In Memory of
Irene Gray
Eric L. Goldson
Thomas White

Contents

Tables

Acknowledgments

This book is the culmination of the efforts and support of many individuals. First and foremost, without the honesty and good faith of the fifty-three young women who participated in this study, there would be no story to tell. I wish to thank those who participated in the Yale AIDS Colloquium Series for their suggestions when this project was still in the early stages. Additionally, several others contributed in many ways throughout this process: the staff at the Yale University Social Sciences Library, as well as members of the Department of Sociology; and my friends and colleagues at Purdue University, especially Dean Knudsen, David Fasenfest, Myrdene Anderson, and Evie Blackwood. At Central Connecticut State University my new colleagues in Criminal Justice, African Studies, Anthropology, and Sociology and Social Work have been very helpful as well. Abigail Adams, Susan Pease, and Evelyn Phillips have shared ideas and data and read drafts of sections of this book. Celina Middleborough and Lorraine Jurgilewicz provided boundless technical support.

I owe a debt of gratitude to others who have guided me through this process: Wendy Battles, Tanya Bennett, Lawrence Biondo, Catha Day Carlson, Mark Harding, Iris Harley, Jeff Harman, Tony Hernandez, Ngadi Kponou, Sandy Masuo, Debbie Phelps, Dina Strachan, and Gary Sullivan; and my mentor and friend, the late Professor Martin U. Martel. To my second family, Lisa Jones Gordon, Rick Gordon, Mathieu, and Jennifer Gordon: thank you. And to my family: Clara Johnson White, Richard T. White, Lorraine White, and Naomi, Javier, Kenneth, and Eudora—you have offered me more than I can say.

My editor Dean Birkenkamp, and Rebecca Hoogs, Editorial Assistant, have been patient and supportive through the entire process.

Finally, I wish to recognize and thank all those men and women who tirelessly devote themselves to bettering the lives of young men and women in our communities. These are the unsung heroes.

Introduction:
To Be Young, Female, and Black

The current AIDS crisis is one that touches on all segments of our society. Regardless of age, gender, race, social class, sexual orientation, or religion, we all have been forced to confront the reality of this disease. Our challenge, both as individuals and as a society, is to find ways to communicate about both AIDS and the virus that precedes it—human immunodeficiency virus (HIV). This is particularly true because AIDS has slowly begun to destroy the lives of many young people, particularly black women.

Young men and women of African and Latino descent have been most affected by HIV and AIDS. Since over fifteen years ago, when the virus was first detected and tracked systematically, these young men and women have found themselves increasingly affected and infected. Why is this the case?

In this book I discuss why HIV has disproportionately infected black adolescents—specifically young women. They are the most likely to carry the virus and to die from AIDS. They are also excessively studied by all sorts of experts hoping to understand their "condition." Many of those engaging in this process of supposed discovery and disclosure do more harm than good; they provide a skewed and negative image of black teenagers, one that presents them as sexually driven, reckless, and fatalistic. Such depictions have done little to contribute to the explanation of what is happening among black teenagers.

Politics, mythology, and fear have affected the substance of research concerning teenage sexual and risk-taking behaviors. For example, little data on HIV and black adolescents concern the specific ways in which adolescents come to think of themselves as sexual beings. Conventional wisdom still dictates that adolescent sexuality is by defini-

1

tion immature and thus need not be studied systematically. Further, the image of blacks as naturally sexual is still pervasive—race is used to explain HIV status.

Adolescence is a developmental stage in which teenagers challenge and redefine their identities. Teenagers are seen as adults in formation. They are encouraged to experiment with social roles, and therefore they are not expected to assume social or fiscal responsibility for themselves. They test others' expectations as well as their own in a search for maturity and adult status. They are confronted with boundaries that define age-appropriate behavior and roles. Sexuality is one of the avenues through which this process of change occurs.

Although we now define adolescence as a transitional period between childhood and adulthood, do all teenagers develop at the same rates? Does a brief period of adolescence help explain why some young women begin sexual activity at such early ages? What do teenagers feel about themselves and their environments, and to what extent does all of this influence their behavior and potentially their risk of contracting a sexually transmitted disease such as AIDS?

Recognizing the effects of environment on teenagers involves considering the way teenagers function within their particular physical and social space. The neighborhood or community is a microcosm of the social order teenagers expect to encounter as adults. Therefore, perceptions of employment opportunities, educational access, violence, and other elements shape what young women expect in their futures. These factors seem to be unrelated to one's sexual behavior. In fact, these factors *are* relevant because they convincingly illuminate both how and why there is variation in reproductive and sexual behavior by both race and class. Sexual activity and reproductive choices do not occur in isolation. A range of social and societal factors shape the process of sexual identity development and sexual behavior. One's circle of friends, relationships with parents, and available role models in the community are all greatly influential in the process of identity development.

Given all of these considerations, the purposes of this book are to present a comprehensive analysis of the sexual behavior of young black women,[1] one that considers this behavior within a larger political, economic, and social context; to determine how AIDS has affected the sexual decision making of young black women; and to suggest how AIDS and sex education programs should more effectively represent what these teenagers need. To address these issues, I will frequently refer to case studies from a series of intensive interviews conducted with fifty-three young women, between thirteen and nineteen years old, who lived in New Haven, Connecticut—a small city.[2]

By making AIDS among black adolescent females the focus of my study, I do two things. First, I consider the ways teenagers experience sex. Second, on the basis of their own observations and experiences I can highlight what their perceptions of AIDS, sex, and reproduction are, as well as how they behave. By studying AIDS and black teenagers' sexuality from a sociological perspective, I illustrate how people develop their sexual identities and how the factors inherent in this developmental process affect how individuals assimilate and react to the AIDS epidemic.

Understanding what young black women experience and what affects their sexual and reproductive lives requires considering two main factors: (1) poverty and economic status and (2) race. Racial-ethnic heritage explicitly shapes the lives of young black women in the United States. At the same time, social class also influences their lives. These factors apply to considerations of sexuality and reproduction, as both race and class affect these matters as well as AIDS risk. Thus, one must address the links between race and class to understand risky behavior as well as to develop effective interventions.

While black women and Latinas are subject to racism and sexism, the reality of their experiences are mitigated through differences in social class background. These differences are exemplified in sexual and reproductive decision making. We can gain a better understanding of what social factors affect black adolescents' sexual and reproductive decisions by considering how economic and other material conditions can shape decision making and behavior.

Sexual behavior and decision making are individualized, personal processes that are affected by social forces. Engaging in sexual behavior and making contraceptive choices are actions grounded in social contexts. What concerns me about the existing literature on teenage sexuality and/or AIDS is that it infrequently includes an analysis of the role sex plays within a given range of options. By defining sex as a private behavior that occurs "behind closed doors," the fact that various social factors underlie sexual behavior may be overlooked. Since sex involves more than biological drive, studying sexual behavior must always include how one is socialized to be a sexual being and how this socialization is manifested in decisions and action. If we accept that sexuality is developed through a social process, then we also need to pay attention to whatever environmental, material, and social factors guide this process of development. Add to this the question of what contraceptives to use and when, and suddenly sex and risk assume different meanings.

Recent research on the sexual behavior of young men and women indicates that youth of color in particular are not taking precautions (whether through contraceptive use or behavioral modification) to reduce the risk of contracting sexually transmitted diseases (STDs). Additionally, some black youth *appear* to be most likely to engage in risky behavior such as frequent sex with random partners, substance abuse, and erratic contraceptive use. The data indicate this trend because black teenagers are more likely to exhibit outcomes associated with risky behavior such as becoming pregnant and contracting a sexually transmitted disease. Because these outcomes are often used to measure rates of risk taking, it seems as if black youth engage in risky activities.

We need new approaches to the study of black sexuality for two reasons. First, there is little research on black women that addresses AIDS and sexuality from a wide-ranging, holistic perspective, in which the entirety of their lives is considered in order to better understand the role sex plays. Second, even less prevalent is research on black teenagers' sexuality and AIDS.

The way we discuss the AIDS crisis is affected by emotional, religious, moral, scientific, and personal elements. Discussing the impact of AIDS on adolescents of all races also involves recognizing these unresolved social issues, stereotypes, and value systems. I feel that it is important to acknowledge these conflicts and to be mindful that the relevance of this project is at least partly defined by the changing tide of a larger discourse about sex and AIDS. We have to continue to talk about AIDS and sex, but, more important, we need to challenge ourselves to take an honest look at the lives of adolescents in our communities. Denial, fear, and silence do nothing more than allow this disease to cut short the invaluable lives of those who comprise our future.

The first chapter outlines the current rates of sexual and reproductive activity, as well as rates of HIV and AIDS infection. In "Picturing the AIDS Epidemic," I discuss the social and biological factors associated with rates of infection. This includes attention to the ways nationwide perceptions of AIDS have changed over time. In chapter 2, "In the City," you will be introduced to the young women from the case studies and interviews I have conducted. The chapter depicts—often in their own words—what their lives are like.

I will then discuss the lessons teenagers learn regarding men, sex, marriage, and AIDS from their friends and family in chapter 3, "Talking to Girlfriends and Family." The ways both intimate and sexual relationships develop and affect the kinds of behavior a young woman will engage in and how she deals with AIDS will be considered in chapter 4, "Building Relationships: Love, Dating, and Romance." All of the themes in these previous chapters will be used to explain the frequency and timing of sexual activity among young black women in the fifth chapter, "Sexuality and Womanhood."

In chapter 6, "Contraception: Safer Sex or Birth Control?" I report on rates of contraceptive and condom use. The ultimate irony is that while teenagers have a more general understanding of what AIDS is, they now overidentify AIDS and mortality with condoms. Thus, in chapter 7, "Ultimate Risk: Perceptions of AIDS and HIV," I summarize what teenagers know about AIDS, HIV, and condoms and what all of this represents for them in their personal lives. In the final chapter, "Just Say No? Reflections on the Reality of AIDS," I tie all of these chapters together with a few thoughts on what we need to do to combat risk among teenagers more effectively. To encourage further discussion, a resource list of agencies and information clearinghouses is provided in an appendix for those in search of additional information.

1

Picturing the AIDS Epidemic

What is it about AIDS that makes it so frightening and upsetting for many of us? Though many financial and scholarly resources are used to study this disease as well as the virus causing it, we seem to conclusively know little about it, and even less about it that we can understand. AIDS continues to be a mysterious presence in, and a potential threat to, all of our lives. It is a deadly disease, one that can live in our bodies for years without our knowledge. The fact that information about AIDS changes so rapidly makes it more deadly. Even so, we often hesitate to learn more about this disease, for that knowledge might require that we challenge many basic assumptions and expectations held very dear to us as a society.

In the following discussion I will describe in more detail just how AIDS has affected our lives. This includes a review of the rates of infection, as well as what rates of infection mean for the future of young black men and women. It is important to review the ways HIV can be transmitted, because this will result in a better understanding of how and why young adults are often susceptible to infection. All of our scientific and more popularly based knowledge of the disease ultimately have shaped the way we talk about and perceive AIDS and HIV.

High-visibility public figures who have acknowledged their HIV or AIDS status have heightened awareness and generated discussion in the media, in classrooms, in homes, at work, and so on. Public discussion has reflected changes in the awareness of and sensitivity to the AIDS crisis. For teenagers in the United States, their feelings about AIDS and what they do in response to these feelings naturally have been influenced by a host of factors.

A second issue also needs to be considered: the way AIDS is studied. Obviously we can only better equip ourselves to slow the rate of infection with access to accurate information. This information comes from biologists, chemists, and others in the health and medical fields as well as from social scientists (such as myself) who investigate the influence of social (environmental, community, psychological/emotional) factors. Research shapes what we all—laypersons and professionals—know about AIDS and how we use the information. To generate a full base of knowledge about AIDS and black adolescents, we need to consider the biological, epidemiological, social, and psychological factors connected to the disease.

HIV and AIDS

The human immunodeficiency virus (HIV) is popularly known as the virus that causes AIDS. This virus can be contracted only by exchanging bodily fluids with a person or substance that already has the virus. Not using condoms during any sexual contact (intercourse, oral sex, and anal sex)[1] with an HIV-infected individual, using a needle already used by someone with HIV, and *on rare occasions* coming into contact with HIV-infected organs and tissues, blood, or blood products[2] put an individual at risk for contracting HIV. Pregnant women who are HIV-positive can pass the virus to the fetus in utero, and breast-feeding women who are HIV positive may pass the virus to their infants.[3] Scientists use the term *at risk* to refer to the possibility that one or more individuals might contract the disease. Anyone who has participated in any of these behaviors is technically at risk.

Not all behaviors carry the same risk. Certain substances contain higher concentrations of HIV and thus are more effective at transmitting the virus. Blood, semen, and vaginal/cervical secretions have very high concentrations of HIV; breast milk has a lower concentration, and negligible traces of HIV have been found in saliva, tears, sweat, feces, and urine. For HIV to be transmitted, the fluid has to come into contact with a body surface that has been broken or cut. This is why intercourse carries such risk—skin breakage/rupture is far more likely because tissue in the vagina and anus is so delicate. Injection drug use is also extremely risky because it involves the purposeful breakage of the skin, and the virus can be introduced directly into the bloodstream. French (deep or wet) kissing is less risky; even though the inside of the mouth and the gums may have cuts, saliva rarely contains HIV.[4]

HIV is an immunosuppressant, which means that it is a virus that weakens a person's immune system, leaving her susceptible to a variety of infections.[5] HIV attacks a person's T-cells—the white blood cells that are necessary for disease resistance. Eventually, opportunistic infections take advantage of a person's weakened physical state, further compromising her ability to fight off future disease. Therefore, HIV is commonly viewed as a virus causing chronic disease—treatable illnesses such as pneumonia, meningitis, and numerous neurological disorders that eventually become unresponsive to drug therapies, thus becoming chronic or recurrent.

According to the Centers for Disease Control (CDC), an individual usually goes through a number of stages once exposed to HIV. In the beginning, her HIV status will go undetected; she will not have been diagnosed. Then, though formally recognized as HIV positive, she will be asymptomatic (show no signs that she may have HIV). In the next stage, her immunological system will begin to shut down. The period during which she is free from symptoms may last from eight to fifteen years, which is why early testing after exposure to any risk is so important. An individual might not know she has been exposed, thus facing the possibility of passing the virus on to many unsuspecting people and lessening the possibility that her quality of life may be maintained.

What distinguishes being HIV positive from having AIDS are a number of health factors that have been formally defined (and are constantly refined) by the CDC, the National Institutes of Health (NIH), and many other federal and national public health organizations. The reason that HIV is considered to result in AIDS is that the virus begins to break down an individual's ability to produce antibodies and to fight off increasingly debilitating disease.[6] Once a person has what are known as AIDS-indicator diseases, and once her white blood cell count falls below a cutoff point, she will be designated as having AIDS.

AIDS is an acronym that stands for acquired immune deficiency syndrome. This more technical term is a very accurate description of the disease. One is formally recognized as having AIDS when a number of the opportunistic infections associated with HIV seem to recur with frequency and when the person exhibits symptoms such as Kaposi's sarcoma (KS), a form of skin lesion often visible to the naked eye; esophageal candidiasis, a form of thrush or infection in the esophagus or throat; and pneumocystis carnii pneumonia, excessive weight loss due to diarrhea, and a T-cell count below 200. What is important to note is that these conditions can be present in a person who is not HIV infected. Therefore, self-diagnosis is impossible and ill advised. Actual diagnosis involves assessing the severity of the illnesses, frequency of infection, T-cell count, along with inquiring into a person's past risk taking, including exposure to HIV-infected individuals.

Recently, public health agencies have recognized that the mode of diagnosis for women is often different than for men. First, certain indicators, such as KS, occur infrequently among women. Furthermore, some diseases are unique to women that must be considered in their formal AIDS diagnosis. Recurring drug-resistant candidiasis, pelvic inflammatory disease (PID), and other specific gynecological conditions such as frequent bouts with sexually transmitted diseases (STDs) are signals to health care providers that they should investigate the possibility of HIV infection and possibly AIDS. Although these symptoms raise the question of HIV exposure, they certainly are not solely associated with HIV and AIDS; they may point to other gynecological problems.

As this review of some of the indicators—or signals—of AIDS shows, people who succumb to the virus do so because their bodies have become unable to battle the repeated onslaught of infectious disease. Each time the body has to fend off an infection, using up precious reservoirs of T-cells and white blood cells, the person is left depleted and therefore more susceptible to additional disease and illness. Although no vaccine or cure exists for this disease, infected persons, especially in the latter half of this decade, have more health care options. Overall healthy living—diet, exercise, stress reduction—is definitely useful. Furthermore, new drugs are available that have been effective for some people living with AIDS. In addition to azidothymidine (AZT), which inactivates the virus, there are protease inhibitors that actually interfere with the virus's ability to replicate. Protease inhibitors are taken along with other immunity-building drugs in what is called a "drug cocktail."[7]

An individual can reduce her risk of infection in a number of ways. First, a latex condom, especially one with nonoxynol-9 (a spermicide that kills HIV), is very effective for protection during oral, anal, and vaginal intercourse. Latex should be used during oral sex with either a man or a woman—a dental dam, actually a square of latex, can be used during oral sex with a woman. For an injection drug user, sharing needles or any component of his works (cooker, water, etc.) is a risky prospect. These are all behaviors to avoid. Providers suggest that breast-feeding women—particularly those with a known risk of exposure—consider bottle-feeding rather than breast-feeding. Another outlet is the HIV antibody test itself. This test is confidential, which means that the results are on a person's health records, but cannot be disclosed to anyone without her permission. Testing for HIV can also be anonymous, which means the person does not even give her name—but is instead identified by a number. Ultimately, what each person can do is to contact a hot line, a clinic, or a heath care provider with questions.

Rates of Infection

Rates of AIDS infection have already reached crisis levels. By the end of 1996, 573,800 persons were reported to have had AIDS.[8] Over 68,000 cases were reported during 1996 alone. Most people living with AIDS (PLWAs) are between thirty and thirty-nine years old. Since 1993, HIV infection has been the most common cause of death among persons twenty-five to forty-four years old: more than 70 percent of people dying from AIDS-related complications were from this age group. In 1996, 41 percent of adults with AIDS were black. Rates of infection are increasing the fastest among young adults—especially among females. In fact, much of the continued rise in heterosexual transmission is due to increases in the rate of infection among young women. The situation is especially bad for many black women and Latinas. Many reported cases are among black women and Latinas in their late twenties—38 percent of black women and 41 percent of Latinas with AIDS are between twenty-five and thirty-four years old.[9] The death rate (due to HIV infection) among black women aged twenty-five to forty-four is nine times as high as the rate among Caucasian women.

Blacks and Latinas constitute approximately 72 percent of females who have tested HIV positive throughout the United States but are a minority of the nationwide population of women (21 percent). This figure means that black women and Latinas are *disproportionately* infected. HIV infection and AIDS rates for women of color are particularly acute in large cities on both coasts. For example, in New York City, AIDS frequently has been identified as the primary cause of death among minority females aged twenty-five to twenty-nine for the past ten years.

Forty percent of adolescent females thirteen to nineteen years old who tested HIV positive between July 1996 and June 1997 contracted the virus through heterosexual contact. An additional 55 percent did not report the mode of transmission of the virus.[10] Fifty-eight percent of HIV-positive black women are between twenty and thirty-four years old. The window for testing HIV positive is usually within six months of contracting the virus and it may be another ten years before testing positive for AIDS.[11] Thus, it is safe to assume that these women may have contracted HIV in their teens and early twenties. Coupled with the reality that most contract the virus through heterosexual contact, these findings illustrate how important it is to pay particular attention to whatever factors affect adolescents' sexuality and how all of this is associated with their exposure to the virus.

A City Faces a Crisis: AIDS Data for New Haven

To understand the current situation faced by black teenage women, we can refer to national statistics that document the path HIV and AIDS have taken within this group of young people. Although this is an important starting point, we also need to be able to investigate HIV and AIDS in even greater depth, which involves considering any and all factors associated with the AIDS crisis among teenagers. One method that makes such analysis more feasible is a case study. By selecting a community or town with a substantial number of teenagers, we can continue exploring adolescence and AIDS. The case study can provide working examples of what might be happening to teenagers in other parts of the United States. It also enables us to raise questions from more individualized vantage points than is possible with large-scale data sets; we can use specific examples to better understand what large studies have found and to think about what the statistics mean for the individual. For the sake of this discussion, we will be considering the stories found in New Haven, Connecticut. Though this city is profiled in detail in chapter 2, a few facts described here will show why it makes an important and instructive city to study in detail.

Connecticut has had more AIDS cases in the past two decades than forty other states.[12] It usually ranks in the top fifteen each year for incidence rates (number of new cases of infection for every 100,000 residents). Some interesting trends are apparent when compared with national averages. For example, female AIDS cases for the state have continued to increase, while the proportion of female cases nationwide has been declining over the past two years.[13] AIDS cases among black women have declined (44 percent) but have remained stable for black men (38 percent).

New Haven residents comprised 17 percent of the state's AIDS cases in 1996. According to one city health department report, 41 percent of people reported to have AIDS were black, 25 percent Latino, and 33 percent Caucasian.[14] New Haven is particularly important to study because of its high rates of teenage pregnancy, as well as STD and AIDS infection. For example, adolescents comprise 4 percent of all reported cases, and adult women comprise 20 percent of the total number of cases. These proportions are about twice the national average. Also, one-third of the state's pediatric AIDS cases (children under two years old) are from New Haven.[15] It should not be surprising to note that a disproportionately high number of reported cases in the Northeast are from New Haven. These findings illustrate the need to address teen sexual behavior in a city such as New Haven, where the reported rate among adolescents is high. If we come to understand what has occurred there, then perhaps the information will be useful in other communities throughout the nation.

The Social and Social Scientific Meaning of AIDS

First and foremost AIDS is known as a disease, one that has defied and challenged the scientific community. But AIDS is also associated with larger social, political, moral, religious, and ethical questions. When we talk about AIDS in the public arena, it is rarely as only a biological or scientific fact. AIDS has caused this nation to deal with many sensitive topics in ways that other diseases, even STDs, has not. Social science research has begun to reflect the changes in broader social debates around sexual behaviors and activities in the AIDS era.[16] When we talk about the social-scientific meaning of AIDS, we refer to the entire debate around it, including the many ways the perceptions of the disease have changed in sociological (or social) terms.

Initially, scientific concern over the HIV/AIDS epidemic focused on gay men, because they were the first to be publicly associated with this disease. In the early 1980s a few newspapers reported on a mysterious disease called a "gay cancer" that was identified in gay men living in New York and San Francisco as well as in parts of Europe. Because they are a marginalized social group, the image of gay men at risk, living with and dying from AIDS, was not of great concern for some people. Because it was still considered a "gay disease," little attention was paid to risk among heterosexuals as a group.[17]

This was a time in the history of AIDS and HIV research when the question of risk of infection was addressed in terms of groups of people. If the virus seemed to cluster, or concentrate, within certain categories of people, the conclusion was that perhaps these same categories faced a higher risk of infection. Risk and risky behavior were defined in terms of certain groups, categories, or communities of people. Anyone who was identified as a member of these risk groups was automatically labeled "high risk." As a result of this assumption, an inordinate amount of attention was paid to gay men as a high-risk group. Although focusing energy on such communities was not necessarily unreasonable, what emerged subsequently derailed the assault on HIV and AIDS.

Gay men became associated with the disease. Gay men constituted a high-risk category because of their sexuality. People began to assume that if a man was homosexual, then he was most likely HIV infected or would eventually test positive. As long as a person was not gay, he was safe from infection. AIDS began to represent more than a health threat: it symbolized issues regarding people's morality. AIDS began to represent, for a few people within and outside of the scientific community, a morality play—a test of people's moral strength and fortitude. While the spotlight was on gay men, the disease began to take a stronghold on other segments of the population: heterosexual men's, women's, and children's rates of infection continued to increase. The global picture of AIDS was also changing. Though the rates of infection in many Eastern European countries and Southeast Asia were exceptionally high, attention turned to the rapidly increasing rates in African and Latin American countries. Residents of these countries became the next groups of people to be defined as high risk by virtue of their nation of origin.[18] Within the United States, the growing rates of infection among blacks and Latinos led to a similar conclusion for some of our own scientists. Attention turned to other risk groups: African and Haitian immigrants had their entry restricted, and black and Latin Americans were also rendered suspect. Thus, the AIDS debate was transformed into one about race, nationality, sexuality, and eventually socioeconomic status (SES).

This approach to the AIDS crisis was increasingly criticized. Many worried that the emerging discourse would enable racially and sexually biased views to flourish. As a result, scientists, policy analysts, members of government, and many others acknowledged that they needed to shift the perceptions of AIDS and HIV. Additionally, public figures, ones respected by many segments of the country, started to acknowledge their HIV-positive status publicly. By the mid-1980s, Rock Hudson had died from an AIDS-related illness. His death contributed to the growing attention paid to AIDS.

Public interest in and concern over HIV increased, and the conceptualizations of transmission began to shift from risk groups to risk behavior. Any number of behaviors could result in infection. Research verified that individuals using injection drugs could pass or contract the virus. Sexual partners eschewing condoms increased their own risk. Pregnant HIV-positive women could infect fetuses, and those who breast-fed would most likely infect their infants.[19] It was no longer valid to divide people into "safe" and "unsafe" categories. High-risk individuals could not be identified by any physical or personality traits. Perhaps, then, others who seemed to belong to a "safe" category might not be safe after all.

Defining and Identifying Risk

What does it mean to claim that individuals are at either a high or low risk for infection? In the case of HIV, because new information is literally discovered every day, perceptions of risk are constantly being challenged and are changing. Concurrent with the realization that adult women and heterosexual men were also at risk of infection was an increasing concern over teenagers. As the number of teenagers becoming pregnant and rates of childbirth indicate, a substantial number of teens are sexually active, and some are also engaging in unprotected sex.[20] Because HIV is contracted through many intimate kinds of activity, this issue of risk is normally defined in terms of who engages in what behavior and how often.

Technically, one incident involving contact with an HIV-infected individual could result in transmission of the virus, but yet some may engage in risky behavior frequently and not become infected (a fact that has generated images of sex in particular as Russian roulette). Given all of these unknowns, what exactly does risk mean in a biological sense? Furthermore, what does risk mean for people on a personal level?

Unprotected sex implies potential exposure to HIV. What is happening among teenagers that explains this persistent risky behavior? Consider what impact AIDS and other sexually transmitted diseases may have on sexual and reproductive decisions for a young woman. To understand behaviors connected with sexual means of transmission among teenagers, we need to know how a teenager's sexuality develops over time, what constitutes risky behavior to her, and how she learns about AIDS and sex. Emphasizing these factors can contribute to a more complete understanding of why young women of color are overrepresented in the cohort of people with HIV, AIDS, and other STDs.

Although the media have brought to public attention stories about Magic Johnson, Arthur Ashe, Rock Hudson, Greg Louganis, Eazy-E, and Ryan White, what relevance do they have for the "average" teenage woman of color? To what extent are these young women influenced by what goes on around them? What are teenagers' perceptions of the disease, and how are these perceptions influenced by environment, family, peers, the media, or psychological/emotional characteristics?

Black Teenagers and Risk

As much of the data collected over the past few years have shown, black teenagers face a high probability of contracting STDs and getting pregnant, particularly in comparison with national statistics. Poor black females in this age group are more likely to become pregnant than middle-class black females. What exactly does it mean to claim that they are at greater risk for all of this, and how accurate are these claims?

Explanations of rates of HIV infection focus on high-risk behaviors—for example, unprotected sex, multiple sex partners, and injection drug use. On the surface, this view would indicate that black teenagers who are infected engage in any one of a number of behaviors: they infrequently use condoms, and/or have many sex partners, and/or use more drugs than other teens. There is, however, more to consider. Unfortunately, what clouds the issue of black youth and risk are a number of false assumptions made by scientists and laypersons alike. Some studies have presented a picture that depicts black teenagers as sexually voracious, irresponsible, and fatalistic.

As the discussion of risk groups showed, identifying a person who engages in risky behaviors can be easily transformed into a discussion about the qualities of that person. We must remember that sexual and reproductive activity, and associated risk taking, does not occur in a social vacuum. A range of social and societal factors shape the process of sexual identity development and sexual behavior. One's circle of friends, relationships with parents, and available role models in the community all greatly influence the process of identity development. Furthermore, the neighborhood or community is a microcosm of the social order teenagers expect to encounter. Perceptions of employment opportunities, educational access, violence, and other elements shape what young women expect in their futures.

These institutional and structural factors are relevant because they provide a context in which to understand race and class variation in reproductive and sexual behavior and related trends in HIV infection. Black women have been, and continue to be, subject to societal barriers because of their race. However, social class position tempers the way black women experience these barriers. Obviously, regardless of social class black women are "seen" as black. At the same time, class affects their lives. In spite of racism, teenagers from middle-class families may be exposed to a social reality at odds with ones faced by poor black teenagers. This more privileged social reality affects how teenagers perceive their lives and how they intend to behave. Young black women share experiences based on race and gender, but they differ because of class. Young women share experiences because of gender and class, but this commonality is tempered by race.

As far as inquiries into risky behavior, social science researchers and the popular press have been guilty of explaining risk among black females as purely the result of racial characteristics—namely, black culture. If one argues that blacks have unique cultural perspectives on sexuality, does this mean that centuries of contact with various ethnicities has had no impact? Or that blacks are different because of some trait associated with their color? It is important to remember that identifying who is at risk is different from identifying *why* people engage in those behaviors in the first place. Determining whether an individual will be at a high risk for contracting HIV requires a creative tactic. Research on the disease needs to investigate other factors that might be associated with engaging in risky behaviors. In other words, considering what places a person at risk requires investigating not only what teenagers do, and with what frequency, but *why* they do what they do. We need to concern ourselves with social factors that might shape the choices available to teenagers.

In terms of understanding risk and risk-related behavior, the growing body of literature concerning AIDS, sexual behavior, and minority adolescents in particular can be separated into three categories. First, there is demographic and epidemiological research. Such studies consider statistical shifts in the incidence of infection (the distribution of disease by categories such as race, gender, region, and age), prevalence (the number of people currently infected), and the rates of sexual activity in the targeted population (see, e.g., the Centers for Disease Control's *HIV/AIDS Surveillance Report*, *Morbidity and Mortality Weekly Reports* [*MMWR*] and AIDS surveillance reports available through most states' Department of Health).[21] These statistics are obtained from clinics, hospitals, and community health centers. Statistics also enable epidemiologists and the like to calculate the likelihood that individuals may contract HIV and AIDS.

A second category of research concerns the accuracy of AIDS/STD, sex, and contraceptive knowledge among respondents and the effectiveness of education and outreach. Surveys and tests document the knowledge base of teenagers. A number of journals, including *Youth and Society*, *Adolescence*, *AIDS Education and Prevention*, *Family Planning Perspectives*, and *Advance Data* (a publication available from the U.S. Department of Health and Human Services) routinely publish such findings.

A popular presumption is that the more teenagers know and the more prepared they are, the less likely they are to expose themselves to risk; that teenagers with more knowledge face a lower risk than teenagers who do not know about AIDS. This assumption poses a problem, however. Because most teenagers who engage in high-risk sexual behavior have at least a rudimentary understanding of how serious HIV is and how it can be contracted, it is apparent that knowledge alone does not result in risk reduction.

Other research, more focused on cultural differences in sexual behavior, depends on either surveys/interviews or participant observation. One vantage point proposes that black teenagers' behavior is culturally determined. Accordingly, risky behaviors are those that are culturally valued and thus rewarded. So, as an example, if black teenagers engage in sexual intercourse more frequently than other teenagers, thus increasing their risk of infection, they may do so because sexuality is culturally valued. There is a long tradition of studies on the lives of blacks and Latinos. Some of this research has contributed to a clearer understanding of racial-ethnic differences.[22] Another body of work, some of it outdated, continues to reinforce or generate racial stereotypes about the social behavior of blacks.[23] Teenagers' sexual behavior is seen as a symptom of either pathology or maladaptation.

Some studies use a more complex and sophisticated position: that one's culture is a combination of race, class, religion, age, ethnicity, geography/region, and other characteristics.[24] Everyone is shaped by a cultural tradition, and none of these traditions is by definition more dysfunctional or maladaptive than others.

As this last category of research shows, there is literature in the social sciences that investigates teenage sexual identity and high-risk behavior from a comprehensive perspective. These studies do not focus solely on the connections among sexual behavior, contraceptive use, and AIDS knowledge. Instead, they have begun to look at the lives of teenagers in totality, and thus attempt to identify the importance placed on sexual behavior within adolescents' lives. For these researchers, teenage sexuality *in and of itself* is not problematic. Even in these projects the findings identify what people do, but not necessarily why they behave in or feel a specific way.

What much of the work on teenagers overlooks is that there are also teenagers who are not sexually active, as well as those who are "responsible" about their sexual behavior. The important question is what distinguishes these two groups from teenagers who do take risks. Explanations can range from external factors (social institutions and group-level influences) such as the influence of school, friends, family, and the economy to individual factors such as self-esteem, personal values, attitudes, and beliefs. In subsequent chapters, we will consider in greater detail research and theories on teenage sexual behavior, attitudes and beliefs, and AIDS. We will begin to unravel the various kinds of risk black teenagers face, how they perceive this risk, what they truly know about AIDS, and to what extent social and psychological factors influence what these teenagers feel and do in their public and private lives.

2

In the City

Environment influences development. This claim, made by sociologists and psychologists, is deceptive in its simplicity. It suggests that the kind of life led by a young woman is directly related to her outlook. Expectations and hopes are shaped while growing up and are to be realized in adulthood. It is of utmost importance that a young woman's entire life experience be considered when trying to understand the decisions she makes and the beliefs she maintains. Obviously, poor teenagers living in cities deal with a set of unique challenges. They are frequently forced to face uncertain futures. Middle-class teenagers' lives are different from those of their low-income peers. Even though their home lives may appear no different than poor teenagers', there are still tangible and intangible opportunities available to them. Young women live in many types of communities, interact with friends and relatives, go to school, work, watch television and listen to music, date, and imagine what their futures will look like. Learning about the importance of sex and AIDS in teenagers' lives requires first understanding what it is like to be a teenager in this ever-changing world.

We live in a world where socioeconomics, race, and gender matter. We are stratified, or ranked, based on these and many other socially defined characteristics. Our social location influences our access to educational, occupational, and economic institutions. What emerges out of this system of social stratification—maintained by racism, economic inequality, poverty, as well as sexism—is a social world in which young black men and women are expected to survive. They learn while very young what it means to be black in the United States and what it means to be male or female. Family, school, the media, and other social institutions teach teenagers how to adapt to, function, and participate in the social world.

19

Social stratification influences not only the quality of a young woman's present lifestyle but also her future. This is most apparent in terms of the continuing differential access to good schools that prepare youth for college and future careers. When you are used to having a quality education and a social network that can provide you with summer jobs, college recommendations, and the like, you expect your future to be filled with opportunity, and behave accordingly.

Race and social class are relevant to the emergent AIDS crisis among teenagers. Black and Latino teenagers in urban areas as well as Caucasian teens in rural areas are at a heightened risk of HIV infection. Why is this so? What is it about life in poverty that might be connected to HIV? Is there anything about the lives of working-class, middle-class, or upper-class youth that is associated with a lowered risk of HIV infection? Posing these questions does not mean that social class determines HIV status but merely that certain quality-of-life characteristics associated with SES might also be related to HIV risk. The question of interest here is whether and how community and social class shape teenagers' risk taking and how they behave in their relationships, and whether community and social class also influence teenagers' perceptions of HIV and AIDS.

Social Class and Community

Observations in this book are to a large extent based on the assumption that sexual and reproductive behavior are affected by racial identity and social class. By making this assumption, I am challenging theories that remove sexuality, reproduction, and sexual identity from the public realm. This removal is often evident when researchers define sexuality and reproduction as domestic, private issues only relevant within the parameters of a relationship. What is erroneous about such an assumption is that the most private behavior is indeed connected with the public social world. In other words, sexuality and reproduction are constructed.

Because the social world affects our perceptions of ourselves and how we behave, it is only reasonable to make the claim that research on individuals is similarly affected by the social world—it is shaped by cultural images, symbols, assumptions, stereotypes, and so on. The study of black teenagers' sexuality has been clouded by a basic flaw: the tendency to confound race with poverty and social class. As Deborah Tolman (1996) notes, "On the body of The Urban Girl, social context becomes confused and confounded with race: she is a girl of color, so she must be poor. . . . She is incapable of delaying gratification, fails in school, does not secure employment, and most of all she is sexually promiscuous."[1] Phenomena that may occur because of structural causes are attributed to race differences. Culture and environment are used as code words that superficially relate to structure when in fact they are allusions to race. Racial encoding of this sort is represented in the packaging of images like the "natural" sexuality of blacks as well as more subtle references to "tendencies" in blacks' behavior.[2] Black Americans' behavior is studied and explained as intrinsically black behavior and therefore deviant.

For those who embrace this type of racial perspective, risky behavior among black teens can be just as easily explained as a cultural fact. This assumption is central to the culture of poverty debate in social science literature. One key outcome of minimizing or negating the importance of social institutions and structures in shaping groups is that criticism of these existing institutions and barriers, such as inequality, racism, and sexism, need not occur.

Poverty, Culture, and the Urban Underclass

Debates concerning the poor are often separated into two broad categories: the culture of poverty and structuralism. Theoretical frameworks developed from the culture perspective posit that something is endemic to the state of poverty that prevents the poor from acting in ways that will liberate them from economic hardship and social isolation. People have to adjust mentally to the state of poverty. They cannot expect institutions to function effectively on their behalf, and so they begin to behave in unproductive ways. Social-psychological factors are at the core of the problems the poor experience.[3] Because these frameworks are used in the study of the urban underclass—typically perceived as black—a troubling picture emerges. In considering the state of poverty, the question is, why are so many black people poor? rather than, Why does poverty persist?

Poor families socialize youth to behave in ways that reflect the values and beliefs associated with this "ghetto subculture." Social behaviors of poor youth are thus viewed as pathological and destructive. In fact, "by permitting low-income people to expect that they need never work . . . [there is] a class of people who remain poor because they feel no obligation to contribute to the larger society and who exhibit high rates of out-of-wedlock births, teen pregnancy, long-term unemployment, criminality and drug use."[4] Because so many of the poor visible in urban areas are black, an additional danger arises in the culture-of-poverty literature of making a link between race and class and sexuality. This perspective is a problem when research is intended to inform social policy.

Structural theorists criticize culture-of-poverty theorists for slipping into race- and class-based reductionism. Structuralists counter culturalists by arguing that social institutions greatly influence the behavior of the poor:

> Propelled by a disappearing local economy, disintegrating community institutions, social isolation, and spatial concentration, a subculture of disengagement has apparently surfaced among some segments of the Black youth populations in central cities around the country.[5]

> Adolescents who feel inadequate and inferior, who are without opportunities for meaningful education and work . . . are at the greatest risk. . . . Many have been socially abused; racism and sexism have limited their access to opportunities that some segments of the population take for granted. . . . Minorities in general simply have less access to information and services.[6]

While institutional barriers limit social mobility and result in poverty, the poor share values and aspirations associated with the "mainstream." As such, what the poor do should be interpreted no differently from middle- and upper-income households. Poor communities coexist with more privileged ones and are as subject to "core" or traditional social codes as any other group. The main difference is that they face barriers to acceptable means of satisfying those expectations. What appear to be negative or risky behaviors might actually be rational responses to the range of options available to those low-income teenagers who lack social supports.

What is particularly valuable about material/structural theory is that it does not incorporate a solely behavioral or cultural analysis of the lives of working poor and poor people. Behavior is shaped by more than an individual's choice to act in a particular way. Access to health care, sex education policies, and counseling are as relevant to the way people behave as are self-identity, emotional maturity, and sex-related knowledge. Angela Davis describes the specter of poverty and class in teenage pregnancy in these terms:

> Pregnancy is a symptom of a deeply rooted structural crisis in the U.S. monopoly-capitalist economy—the reverberations of which are being felt most acutely in the Afro-American community. There is a direct correlation between the unprecedented rates of unemployment among Black teenagers and the rise in the birthrate among Black women under twenty.[7]

Any discussion of the effects of poverty is sure to be filled with contradictions. Low-income families are excluded from opportunity, yet often maintain "mainstream" or "traditional" expectations.[8] High rates of pregnancy and STD infection exist among poor teenagers. Exclusion from socially sanctioned access to institutions results in social isolation and alienation. What emerges from all of this? Robert Staples (1986) observes:

> We learn to trust before we learn to love. . . . The members of lower-class families can commit themselves to persons, especially the mothers to their offspring and the siblings to each other; *but they cannot commit themselves to a society they have never learned to trust.* Thus, *the retreatist behavior of the lower class may be a manifestation of the absence of trust* rather than a rejection of social organization in favor of social disorganization.[9]

The Economy and Black Adolescent Life

Economics determine in large part the quality of life available to a teenager. Within the past decade or so, young adults have been faced with a very different social and economic reality than the one encountered by even their older siblings, let alone their parents. High school and college dropout rates are very high. Because of the shifting economic and occupational base in the United States, many young adults who do finish college will return to their parents' homes to live. People are being retrenched and laid off in historic numbers, highly trained older professionals are competing with younger employees for entry-level positions, and the cost of living is higher than ever in many cities.

An increase in the number of black youth in urban cities coupled with a decline in the number of jobs available in primary and secondary labor markets[10] have resulted in adverse conditions for teenagers.[11] Communities do not look the way they used to. In parts of the Northeast and Midwest, previously thriving cities are on the brink of bankruptcy. Cities such as East St. Louis, Illinois, were at some point placed in receivership—forced to look for governance from outside sources. Towns reliant on factory employment are devastated by the movement of business to smaller, more affordable towns in the Southwest and on the West Coast.

The shifting economy hits low-income teenagers the hardest. They are faced with making difficult decisions. This point is especially true for those youth who are partly or solely responsible for their families' financial survival. Although many teenagers report wanting jobs and being frustrated with the minimum wage, a subset reject traditional sources of income and look elsewhere. Other kinds of employment (mostly extralegal or short-term/under-the-table jobs) are readily available and pay well. In depressed conditions, such underground economies replace lost labor markets. The effects of the drug trade on communities, families, and individuals cannot be denied. Conventional sources of employment either are nonexistent or have not paid off, and residents need money.

Black teenagers are aware of the value placed on economic success and social position. They also realize that education and prestigious jobs are the traditional means of attaining this success. However, in the absence of these opportunities (due to the combination of racial discrimination, poor educational opportunities, and gender discrimination), poor black teens may be susceptible to riskier options because of societal pressure to be successful. In spite of these pressures, many poor teenagers *do* resist the lure of these risky opportunities because of other intervening factors, such as family expectations and social support from community members. Whether or not they participate in illicit activity, poor teenagers are hyperaware that their opportunities are limited, and thus their futures may be challenging. Vonnie McLoyd and Debra M. Hernandez Jozefowicz have linked adolescents' expectations with their perceptions of current economic stability within the family.[12] What this means is that young adults who have already experienced a certain amount of economic hardship and who do not believe educational advancement leads to a better economic future expect to have children young, marry young, and get divorced.

This finding is interesting because it raises a basic question: As economic and social conditions for youth worsen, will their expectations of the future be negatively affected as well? Tracing the body of work focused on the lives of low-income black youth provides some answers to this question. A series of books depicts the lives of young black adults in the late 1960s and 1980s and persuasively illustrates the influences of community and urban living on teenagers. Four of the most recent ones—*When Children Want Children* (1989) by Leon Dash, Elijah Anderson's *Streetwise* (1990), *There Are No Children Here* by Alex Kotlowitz (1991), and Terry Williams's and William Kornblum's *The Uptown Kids: Struggle and Hope in the Projects* (1994)—provide very clear examples of the importance of understanding the social context in which a child is raised in order to understand what decisions he or she is likely to make. For example, in *Streetwise*, Anderson describes the shifting status of elders in the community he studied:

[T]he old head served as an important link to the more privileged classes.
. . . Through his example, he offered support to both the local and the

wider systems of social stratification and inspired his boys to negotiate them through legitimate means. Today, as the economic and social circumstances of the urban ghetto have changed, the traditional old head has been losing prestige and credibility as a role model. One of the most important factors in this loss is the glaring lack of access to meaningful employment in the regular economy, resulting in more and more unemployed and demoralized black young people.[13]

As Anderson goes on to show, changes in the urban setting actually do influence how youth are socialized by shifting and constraining the choices available to them. The continual worsening of economic conditions has both a progressive and a cumulative effect on teenagers. They know *how things used to be,* and they are aware of how profoundly they can be affected by slight changes in the job market in which they and their parents participate. How, then, does teenagers' awareness of the reality of life in poor and middle-income urban areas affect the ways they interact with each other and how they develop intimate relationships?

For young black women, including the ones introduced in this book, societal (urban and community) elements affect their sexuality as well as the importance they place on having children, using contraception, and developing intimate relationships. A day in the life of a young woman involves negotiations, compromises, and barriers that emerge from this combination of social factors. The stories found in New Haven point to the realities of life for middle class, working class, and poor black teenagers.

The City Landscape

New Haven is a city located in Connecticut with, according to the Department of Health, 123,893 people in 1996.[14] It has lost 5.04 percent of its population since 1990. The most common image of urban cities—particularly poor ones—is of a large black and Latino population. The racial composition of New Haven, however, is 53.9 percent white, 36.1 percent black, 13.2 percent Latino, and 2.4 percent Asian. The city consists of a few commercial areas, and neighborhoods that range from very wealthy to very poor. Most of the residential areas are racially segregated, except for the neighborhoods where college students live. Yet even these neighborhoods are not racially balanced; they are predominantly white. New Haven has faced financial problems for many years, as evidenced by the state of the main commercial district, where businesses can be short-lived. Some storefronts are vacant, and new "going out of business" sale signs can be spotted daily. Only one street in particular is a busy commercial area; it has a shopping mall and an eight-story office building, bookstores, nationally known specialty stores, small shops, and more than fifteen restaurants.

A small park is also in the commercial area. Many of the city buses run by one corner of this park. On any given school day crowds of youth converge there, often stopping for a snack from one of the neighboring restaurants. Part of Yale University's campus is near the park, and it comprises four to five square blocks of this area. Because of its location, Yale is accessible to many shops that cater to the needs of its students. The variety of businesses is surprising, even for a college community, because this is a relatively small city.

Yale University and the affiliated hospital are the two largest employers in the city, employing 13,300 individuals between them. The third and fourth largest employers are the telephone company and a second hospital, which respectively employ 4,993 and 2,880 people. Management and administrative-level employees live outside New Haven in suburban towns whereas food service, clerical, and "traditional" blue-collar workers live in the city.

Income, Education, and Employment

The 1990 census reported the median household income for New Haven as $25,811.[15] In absolute terms, this number sounds reasonable. However, when income is compared with state averages, another image emerges. The city's median income was 61.9 percent of the state median. In 1995, the per capita income for the city was $12,968, which was 64.2 percent of the state average.[16] New Haven was ranked 163 out of 168 cities and towns based on per capita income. Approximately 21 percent of all persons in the city lived well below the poverty level (these households report an annual income less than $10,000). Project LEAP (Leadership, Education, and Athletics in Partnership) has tracked data for certain neighborhoods in New Haven.[17] Based on census, Department of Labor, and Housing Authority findings, the poverty level in the most hard-hit neighborhoods range from 37.1 to 58.4 percent. When compared with the state poverty rate of 6.8 percent, the implications of life in poverty for some New Haven residents cannot be ignored.

The unemployment rate in New Haven for December 1997 was a low 5.3 percent.[18] However, the picture is drastically worse in certain neighborhoods, where the effects of unemployment are overwhelming. Although slightly older, certain statistics make clear how neighborhoods can vary in terms of unemployment. In 1995, specific neighborhoods in New Haven reported unemployment rates between 31.3 and 85.5 percent.[19] Over the past decade, the unemployment rates have been double to quadruple the city average in a few neighborhoods, where the residents are predominantly black and Latino. Families most affected are female-headed ones, in which children under age of eighteen live. In fact, 40 percent of all children in New Haven live below the poverty level, and 41 percent of female-headed households have annual incomes below the poverty level.

Variation continues in the quality of education residents receive. The majority of all school-age children's reading and math skills fall well below the state average; by late adolescence, youth test at a seventh-grade reading level and a fourth-grade math level. The dropout rate for high school students is almost 40 percent,[20] among blacks the rate is currently 64 percent. Both of these rates are far greater than the state-wide average. Adults do eventually complete their high school education: seven out of every ten adults have either high school diplomas or general equivalency diplomas (GEDs).

These findings help clarify why a city with such a high level of high school educated adults can still have some extremely poor, under-employed communities. Between educational challenges and layoffs (targeting unskilled and semiskilled jobs) reported by three out of the four main employers in the city, it is no surprise that so many black and Latino teenagers, whose parents are greatly affected by these shifts, are growing up poor and working class. This economic and class stratification is to some extent defined by racial-ethnic terms as well. One clear example of this stratification is in housing and residential segregation.

Race and Class in the Neighborhood

Within New Haven a great deal of extensive inequality and stratification among residents is evident. Economically, most of the poor are people of color and are isolated in certain regions of the community. These areas are easily identified by the lack of public works and by the deterioration of property. Commercial traffic is concentrated in some of these areas because they are the sites of major thoroughfares. Although residents are socially and politically isolated from the rest of the city, their neighborhoods represent shortcuts used by commuters to access other sections of the county.

Most Latino families live in the poor and working-class neighborhoods in the city or in other towns outside New Haven. In these areas the businesses tend to be Latino owned and offer products not easily found throughout the rest of the city. About one-fifth of the neighborhoods in New Haven are predominantly black and either working-class or poor. Among the more striking characteristics of New Haven is that even in the poorer neighborhoods there are large single- and multiple-family homes that are at least sixty or seventy years old. Some have been identified as historical sites or as classic examples of the Victorian architecture unique to the area.

Two neighborhoods alongside Yale University and Albertus Magnus College's boundaries contain a substantial number of student, staff, and faculty residences. Wealthy Caucasian families also live in these neighborhoods; their homes are very large, and the streets relatively quiet. There is one black, solidly middle-class community. It is located on the other side of town, surrounded by a number of low-income black neighborhoods.

One area has been the site of increasing racial tensions over the past few years because of a city initiative to build affordable single-family homes for families (many of them black) currently living in Section 8 housing. Some of the largest housing developments are found on the boundaries of New Haven; these are multiple-unit buildings where many of the city's poor and working poor residents live. A few are located in comparably isolated spaces, not easily seen from the main thoroughfares. Plots of land remain untended by their owners and are the areas where cars, large appliances, and pieces of furniture are abandoned.

Youth in the City

The picture painted of many of the 11,183 teens in New Haven appears grim at first glance. Almost half of the people under eighteen years of age live below the poverty level, and an alarming number never finish high school. Although most do not regularly engage in extralegal activities, the police report that the number of those who do is slightly increasing.[21] There is the ever-present temptation for all poor teens to participate in the drug trade (as small-time dealers, runners/messengers) in order to make extra money for themselves and/or their families. They are clearly aware of the tension that exists between attaining the "American Dream" of financial success and the institutional barriers to realizing this goal through legal channels. One English literature teacher at a local high school regularly faced the challenge to be a role model for youth of color, for youth who were fully aware of the economic realities faced by others in the community. She recounted one of her attempts to encourage her students to finish school and seek full time employment:

A group of kids were talking about Tyrell's[22] (a recent high school drop-out) new car. He had just bought a black BMW and had it totally detailed. He paid cash, upfront, in full. I had seen him maybe two weeks ago in a different car that looked brand new. It became obvious that he was doing something bad—how many seventeen-year-olds go around buying new cars every few weeks? . . . So, I tell them that if they get their diplomas and work hard, they can buy cars too. Then this one kid asks me if I finished college. I tell him yes and he asks me what kind of car I drive. You've seen my car, right? [laughs] I drive that Civic. They've seen it too. Case closed. That boy makes more in one week than I make in months. And I'm telling these kids to work at Popeye's or something.

Youth and Violence in the Community

As a result of so many conflicting pressures, it would be easy to imagine untold numbers of junior high– and high school–aged youth becoming involved in criminal activity. The same low-income areas that are home to many black and Latino teenagers are also home to a variety of gangs, some for teens, others for individuals ranging in age from preadolescents to adults. Two have been the focus of a great deal of attention. Both have been embroiled in turf wars with other gangs and, according to some young women interviewed, regularly resort to semiautomatic weapons to resolve territorial disputes. The problem faced by the New Haven police concerning control over gang-related activity is ever present.

Kids will join gangs as a way to make money through criminal activity, but most seem to do so for self-preservation. "Multiple marginality" is the phenomenon that underlies most gang activity.[23] Families are inundated with fiscal problems, neighborhood schools are suffering—youth living in a context where social control has weakened are prime candidates for gang membership. Their peers will protect them and their family. Unfortunately, people are dying because of ongoing violence in their neighborhoods. Teenagers reported regular gang-related conflicts near their schools or in their neighborhoods. One young woman described being shot in a turf battle and not realizing her injury until someone told her she was bleeding. Hearing gunshots was common enough to be ignored.

In a survey of sixth, eighth, and tenth graders in New Haven, 46 percent of students reported having witnessed at least one stabbing or shooting.[24] According to the *Sourcebook of Criminal Justice Statistics* (1996), in 1994 teenagers between sixteen and nineteen had the highest estimated rate of victimization due to crimes of violence. Additionally, in households with annual incomes less than $7,500, most rates of victimization are noticeably higher than other income categories.[25] Witnessing or experiencing physical violence and enduring emotional violence can influence young adults' view of their individual value and affect the way they develop relationships.[26] Violence is a symptom of preexisting challenges faced by residents of the community where such contact is commonplace.

Working Teenagers

Youth from all racial-ethnic backgrounds work after school and on weekends to earn spending money and to offset household expenses. Teenagers work in fast food establishments as well as in small restaurants, coffeehouses, and shops. As one young woman noted, "As soon as one of them shuts down, another restaurant is opening up somewhere and looking for work." Additionally, employers are hiring teenagers for clerical or secretarial assistance.

Unfortunately, in the current economy property taxes and a decline in consumers' purchases have led to an increase in bankruptcies and business relocations.[27] Teenagers have thus faced a weak labor market. Both teenagers and their parents continually voice frustration over the economic state of their community. They believe that they are repeatedly discriminated against on racial and class grounds. Having spoken with some of the parents, many of whom are also in search of new or better jobs, I heard this concern clearly.

> I know how this works. We are always the last to hear about openings, and the last to get hired because they don't want us.

> My kid needs a summer job, so we go to the hospital. We heard that they need help in the cafeteria. She fills out a form and gives it to the woman in personnel. On our way out I just happen to turn around, and see her throwing the form in the trash.

> You know to never put your real address down, 'cause if you do you'll never hear from them again.

Even middle-class youth faced problems when looking for work. Racism affected them as well. But with a different set of social contacts that fostered networking, they had less resistance. Also, they faced a slightly better chance of finding higher paying jobs because employers presumed that they were "safe" teenagers.

> I went to apply for this one job, and the guy told me that there weren't any openings. Now, I knew that wasn't exactly true because my neighbor had told me that they were looking for tons of folks, and I went in the

morning they started looking for people. I went elsewhere and everything turned out okay.

My mother works for the schools. I'm always hearing about work because she's always bugging people for a job for me! It's embarrassing, though.

This group of young women also face challenges. However, they are markedly less suspicious of the dependability of "the system." They believe that eventually they will find work, if necessary.

Sexual Activity and Parenthood

Although they have no standardized means for tracking rates of sexual behavior (as opposed to contraceptive use, pregnancy, and birthrates) for youth in New Haven, social workers, school counselors, clinic staff members, and teachers tend to agree on what is likely to be occurring among teenagers and, more specifically, young women. Some of them estimate that as many as 90 percent of all teenagers by the age of eighteen may have had at least one sexual encounter. The number of teens engaging in regular sexual behavior is most likely one-third to one-half of this (35 to 45 percent). Some report that their teenage clients use contraceptives irregularly and engage in other behaviors that increase the chance of becoming pregnant and contracting STDs.

Most teenage mothers are fifteen to nineteen years old. The birthrate for black teenage females is twice the rate for white teenagers. One predominantly black and Latino neighborhood has frequently led the city with the greatest number of births and the largest percentage of teenage mothers. These high pregnancy and birthrates are cause for concern because they mean that the young adults may have exposed themselves to HIV. This is particularly true in the low-income neighborhoods of color, where the teen birthrates are well above the citywide rate.

Another indicator of risky behavior among both adolescents and adults is the rate of STD infection. Within New Haven, there is a disproportionate number of residents who are HIV positive. By February 27, 1998, New Haven reported 18.53 percent of all cases throughout the state.[28] Sixty-three percent of adults with AIDS are black and 16 percent Latino. For black adults the rate is much higher than their population composition (36.1 percent). For Latinos the rate is proportionate to their citywide population rate of 13 percent. Because few teenagers have full-blown AIDS, the city's surveillance report collapses most adolescent and adult data into one category. Those between twenty and twenty-nine comprise approximately 17 percent of all reported cases.

Rates of other STD infection, a strong indicator of potential HIV infection, can be measured among teenagers. Consequently STD incidence rates are used to calculate the likelihood of HIV infection among
teenagers. The rate of syphilis infection is seventy times higher for
black teenagers than for white ones. Gonorrhea infection is almost
sixty times higher among black teens than among white ones. Thus,
the Connecticut Department of Health has identified that black adolescents are more likely to contract HIV than other racial-ethnic groups.

Teenagers from all racial-ethnic backgrounds engage in a range of
high-risk behaviors, from drug and alcohol use to unprotected sex and
sex with multiple partners. Some of the potential negative results of
these behaviors are clearly illustrated in the findings provided by the
city and state heath departments: unwanted pregnancy, STD infection,
addiction. Those most at risk for these outcomes are black. Though the
different rates of risky behavior by gender are not as readily available,
at the very least we can understand that young women face the risk
of pregnancy in addition to the other physical, social, and emotional
outcomes of these behaviors.

The Lives of Young Black Women

Learning about teenage sexuality involves understanding what it is
like to be an adolescent. Naturally, the young women I have met differ
in terms of their specific experiences, but in some areas their lives were
strikingly similar.[29] Teenagers still deal with dating pressures and expectations that they will be sexually experienced; they sometimes
drink or use other chemical substances; they have love-hate relationships with their parents, relatives, and guardians; they are consumed
with concern about image, reputation, and respect. How different,
then, are they from teenagers in past eras?

Erica, a white case manager at a local social service agency, has lived
in New Haven for many years. She is a single parent, raising a daughter from a previous relationship with a black man. In her line of work,
she has been in contact with young women who are struggling with
identity issues and has observed a remarkable transformation in what
they experience over the last decade. The advent of crack and crack
cocaine, along with other highly addictive state-of-the-art drugs has
damaged some of her clients' home lives. These teenagers have lost
parents to drug addiction, whether through overdosing or through incarceration for illegal activities (a means of supporting their habit).
These girls and young adults have to maintain their households and
often support younger siblings with the help of other relatives.

Even middle-class teenagers, in her view, deal with more stress. They might have financial security, but they, too, live in a more violent world where it is not uncommon to be shot for stepping on someone's Air Jordans (Nike sneakers) or for looking at someone too long. She notices an increased cynicism about their world; they have witnessed businesspeople opting for dishonesty as a way to "get ahead," the divorce rate continuing to rise, men and women remaining one paycheck ahead of poverty, and the continuing challenge to address racism, sexism, and poverty in cities. As others have already argued, teenagers are growing up faster than ever. "[A local program for youth at risk] is trying to fill the gap made by the lack of family structure and the negative influence of schools," Erica says. "Parents often are not around and don't care. There's no one to monitor what's happening, to advocate for kids. Now few kids have even one parent. They live alone, with one partner, in a shelter, etc. Or the parent is using or selling." One special education teacher, who has worked with teens for at least twenty-five years, observes:

> Kids' problems must not, and cannot, be viewed in a vacuum. They take place within a broader context. A child who is a "discipline problem" in the classroom might be acting out frustrations from his home life, or dealing with pressures from friends. Sending him to detention or suspending him will merely be a Band-Aid solution. It does not deal with the root problem, which is more often than not quite complex and extends well beyond his school.

In conversations, it became apparent how aware young women are about their world and their parents' world. Perhaps living in a period when mass communications provide them with a split-second, bird's-eye view of changes in the world combined with the kind of self-consciousness unique to adolescence partly account for this.

Yvonne

One of the young women I met, Yvonne, exemplifies this self-awareness. She is seventeen, goes to school, and lives near the New Haven Health Clinic. She has three younger siblings aged seven, ten, and eleven. Her father disappeared years ago, and her mother is addicted to cocaine and works intermittently as a prostitute. Yvonne works at a grocery store a few mornings of the week and at McDonald's most late afternoons.

Because of her work schedule, Yvonne ran into trouble with her school and ended up in a part-time program for at-risk youth, being identified as a high risk for dropping out. Even with her schedule, Yvonne maintains a B average, intends to go to college, and wants to be a writer. She won an essay contest, which has intensified her interest. When asked to describe her neighborhood, she offered this assessment:

> No one does anything there. Most guys and girls just want to hang out and mess around. Like, see, there's nothing to do except screw with each other. Or get doped [high]. The streets are nasty 'cause they never pick up the trash or sweep the streets. If this was by Morocco Street, it would be different because they have money. It would look pretty cool. Okay, so, like nothing ever works in my house and our landlord won't fix stuff because, you know, who cares about us anyway? I'm just tired of it all; I want to get out.

She later explained that other kids on her block think she is too smart and want her to fail.

According to her counselor, the dealers know her family situation, and some are pursuing her. Because she is strong in math and does not use drugs, she would make an ideal girlfriend for them; she could help with bookkeeping and not be bribed by rival drug dealers who often exchange drugs for information. Yvonne is constantly looking for money to support her family and has admitted that she would do virtually anything for it. She is aware of what these men see in her and is trying to negotiate while not becoming sexually involved with them.

Yvonne has been involved in three or four "long-term" relationships, each one lasting an average of four months. When she was thirteen, Yvonne had her first boyfriend, who was twenty-one. She was not a virgin at that time because she had been raped at ten by one of her mother's "dates" (clients). She did not call this assault rape. In her view it was "another example of some man wanting what he couldn't have . . . he just lost his mind for a while."

Chris

Chris's situation is different, but she is equally aware of the need to compromise and negotiate to survive. Her parents have been married for twenty-two years; her father is assistant principal at her high school, and her mother is a social worker. They live a comfortable middle-class lifestyle in a nearby New Haven suburb where they are one of a small number of black families. She has two part-time jobs, is an A student, and plans to attend college in the fall. She misses her old neighborhood and worries about the impact of their integrated area on her thirteen-year-old sister, Mary.

They [former neighbors] watched out for us, we couldn't get away with anything. Not that I minded. We'd hang out on the porch, where we could see everyone and everything. Now we are in _____, and it just is not the same. It is dead here. Where are the folks? Mary hasn't had the good experiences I had. I know my parents want us to have it better than they did, and I know that moving here is a sign of success, but what are we giving up in return? She [Mary] is good in school, like me, but she hasn't got a lot of black friends. That's messed up. You hear about all these middle class people moving out of the neighborhood and forgetting where they came from. Enough people think I'm acting white as it is. This certainly don't—I mean, doesn't—help things.

Chris is equally concerned with fitting in among her peers and maintaining her strong school record so that she can secure an academic scholarship for college. She is aware of the potential contradictions and pressures that come with these goals. Even so, she is committed to her image as a positive black role model, even if it results in her being less popular with some teenagers. She is acutely aware that her social class has affected how others perceive her racial identity. She is obviously concerned as well about how people will treat her sister.

Chris has dated infrequently, partly because of her parents' influence and partly because she consciously chose to avoid it. As the product of devout Baptist parents (one grandfather is a minister), she was raised to refrain from sexual activity until after marriage. Furthermore, as she has observed, "some of these boys are really pitiful. They spend too much time posturing and not enough trying to do anything better with themselves. I have no time for that, you know." Her education and eventual employment are very important to her; anyone who does not support this goal is "a real waste of time."

LaTasha

At 5' 10" tall, LaTasha is used to people asking her whether she plays basketball: "I wish I were good at it, so I could maybe get a scholarship to college." LaTasha's wish comes from having realized that the likelihood of her going to a competitive college is slim.

LaTasha's parents both work out of the city, on a factory line. They were lucky to get the job because the ratio of applicants per job slot was very high. These new jobs were to mark a turning point in the lives of LaTasha and her two younger siblings: a move to a different neighborhood with a magnet high school. Unfortunately, the expense of the commute to school diminished this possibility.

LaTasha works three afternoons a week after school and during a few weekends. Her boyfriend, who is in his twenties, occasionally gives her money to get her hair and nails done. LaTasha and her boy-friend have been sexually active "Since the beginning" and use contra-ception "most of the time." She plans to marry him once she finishes high school so that she can "start having a decent life, like other peo-ple." LaTasha spoke often of going to college but never indicated any specific plans for attending. When asked to be more precise about col-lege, she said:

> Look, some people aren't meant for college. That's me. I'm just not ready for it. I'm not dumb or anything like that—just don't see the need. What can college give me that a job can't? Money? A nice place? Clothes? You gotta get serious.

Future plans included marriage and children, but not additional edu-cation or a career. She was not even vigilant with birth control because "it wouldn't be a crime to start a family now."

Making Connections: Race, Class, and AIDS

Among the many lessons to be learned in this case study of a city is that being a teenager, regardless of class background, involves more challenges than in past generations. Violence, drug use, sexual assault, unemployment, and sexually transmitted diseases coexist in teens' lives with having crushes on peers, dreaming of the future, socializing with friends, and indulging in dress and fashion distinct to adolescents · in major cities. However, structural conditions do differentially affect the experiences and options available to young men and women, espe-cially teenagers who also deal with racism and discrimination.

Community, environment, and social groups shape us both socially and psychologically. The social world provides conflicting messages that are particularly confusing for teenagers. This social world also of-fers resources for dealing with these conflicts—ones that are often in-adequate and erratic for poor teenagers. Teenagers therefore find them-selves coming of age amid many confusing, frightening, and exciting social currents. What we must now turn to is the implications of all of this on risky behavior and AIDS. This shift in perspective requires recognizing a simple fact. HIV infection occurs because of actions and behaviors, but these actions are influenced and shaped by both social and psychosocial factors. For teenagers, this means facing and adjust-ing to all of these socially determined facts and making decisions based on what they see and what sources (social and emotional) are available to them.

3

Talking to Girlfriends and Family

A few years ago, a song by the hip-hop group Salt-n-Pepa called "Let's Talk about Sex" was popular. This song generated a maelstrom of controversy, for it was perceived as pro-sex, pro-condoms, and thus too dangerous for its teenage listeners. Public response among many adults was negative. The fact that the song appeared to give advice to its listeners, and to encourage discussion, was apparently troubling. Why was the endorsement of sexually responsible communication and discussion perceived as irresponsible in the press? This controversy does show that as a society we might be of at least two minds when it comes to talking about sex and sexuality. On the one hand, the presumption is that someone is to be responsible for educating young men and women. On the other hand, most of the likely parties—parents and mentors, teachers, and public figures—have been made uncomfortable by the task. Some of those who have attempted to assume this responsibility have been met with resistance (anyone from former Surgeon General Joycelyn Elders to the producers of MTVs "Sex in the 90s" series).

Evidently, the debate regarding the appropriate "messenger" for such sensitive information continues. Using this as a starting point, we need to consider in greater depth how young women learn about romance, dating, love, sex, and the outcomes of these experiences. If a parent or elder does not discuss these issues with a young woman, then who does? To whom does she go with her concerns and worries? Lastly, the final challenge is to develop new—or at least effective—ways to encourage discussion and develop ties between young women and those who comprise their support network.

There is a wealth of information about the roles friends and family play in the lives of young adults. One perspective perpetuated by political figures and the popular media is that parents and family are solely

37

responsible for molding children and teenagers. Parents are responsible for teaching youth how to be productive, healthy, and positive individuals.[1] This argument is superficially persuasive: parents introduce children to the "rules of the game," how to negotiate the world. Parents *do* select the neighborhood in which children are raised, the school(s) they attend, and perhaps the church in which they worship. Placing responsibility squarely on the parents' shoulders is unrealistic, however. Although adult role models, mentors, and caretakers provide the framework in which children are to develop, many other social factors influence the attitudes and behaviors of youth.

Once children and teenagers venture into the world on their own, other kinds of social contacts and relationships take hold. As teenagers move through life, they are learning new things, altering their perceptions of their surroundings and relationships, and trying to figure out their roles in the world. This is all part of the process of socialization, through which individuals come to know and understand their world and learn how to survive in it. As we are socialized—by family, school, media, friends, and elders, for example—we are introduced to the rules and norms that regulate the ways we are to function as members of society. In terms of sexuality and intimacy, this implies that how we behave and the decisions we make have been influenced to some extent by others in our environment. Understanding this process means we can neither idealize nor romanticize the influence of family, peers, or any one social institution because they are all interconnected. We all learn about dating, sex, love, and other intimate matters from a wide variety of sources.

Young women are as greatly affected by what people do not say or do as they are by explicit attitudes and behaviors. The relationships they maintain with parents and friends are complex and multifaceted. Therefore, it will be helpful to discuss the influences of family, peers, and to a lesser extent the media on young women. I will also describe the ways young women talked about personal and intimate issues. To whom is a teenage female likely to go if she has a personal problem or a question about sex and AIDS? What messages will she absorb from those in her life, and how will she apply these messages to her own experiences? A commonly held view is that young adults and teenagers do not engage in in-depth discussions about such intimate issues. But that belief is not accurate.

Someone to Talk To

From whom do girls learn about sex? I asked many young women that question. A majority assumed that kids and teenagers learn from their peers. "I figure that kids are going to get the best look from other kids," Sheree observed. "I guess it starts with showing boys your thing, or seeing something you're not supposed to, or something like that. Then you go talk with your girlfriends and swap information." Christiana agreed with Sheree: "When you're a little kid, you probably not going to run to moms to ask about boys, but you will go to your girlfriends probably." Both Sheree and Christiana reflect conventional wisdom as well as what some research on this issue has indicated. According to one study of individuals under seventy years old, "parents were never cited as a primary source of sexual knowledge."[2] In fact, younger adults talked with friends the most and were slightly more likely to approach a teacher with questions about sex than their parents.

This kind of information should cause us to raise questions about the kinds of relationships teenagers have with adults and friends. Although research on the influence of family and friends on youth continues to grow, much of it may not be relevant to black teenagers; it is often based on white youth. What such research has overlooked is that findings concerning white teenagers may not be applicable to black youth. One team of researchers noted, "There has also been considerable interest in the black family generally, but . . . little is known about the adolescent's relationships within it. Our knowledge about the friendship patterns of black in contrast to white adolescents is even more limited."[3]

Because of this lack of information, the perception of black teenagers' relationships can be narrow and stereotypical. If the experiences of black youth differ from those of Caucasian youth—who are considered the norm—black teenagers then will be perceived as experiencing more problems. This view is reflected in the writings of some scholars in family studies, who claim that black youth are often at a disadvantage because they are supposedly raised in deficient households. *Deficient* is defined as female headed, low-income, and urban. Presumably, being raised in such environments means that black teenagers are less likely to develop intimate, gender-appropriate, and supportive ties with either family or friends:

> What is unique to the study of black adolescents is the extent to which being black and adolescent has come to be viewed as synonymous with a variety of social problems. . . . Black youth are monolithically portrayed as urban, low-income, plagued by a multitude of problems, and lacking the resources and/or motivation to effect change in their lives . . . we have learned relatively little about issues of motivation, personality and psychological development, cognitive and moral development, identity

and self-esteem, attitude formation, family relationships with parents and siblings, family socialization issues—in short, issues for which there exists an established and burgeoning literature regarding white youth.[4]

Terms such as culture and environment are frequently used to explain what is supposedly wrong with black youth and their families.

Consider, for example, Daniel Patrick Moynihan's still-controversial 1965 study *The Negro Family: The Case for National Action*. He sought to understand the existence of "nontraditional" family structures and behaviors within the black community. He viewed female-headed households, crime in black communities, and substance abuse as somehow indigenous to black culture. Thus, he identified the cause for these social problems in the very fabric of black families and how they socialize youth. Obviously, past and present research that depicts black family influences on teenagers in this light are troubling in the way they perpetuate negative, stereotypical imagery. What research exists that is relevant to relationships maintained by black youth, and how applicable is this work to the lives of black teenage females in particular?

Teachings about Womanhood: Mothers, Fathers, Aunts, and Sisters

Within the family and community, role models and mentors teach teenagers about the appropriate ways to interact and socialize with others. Parents try to prepare daughters for the real world, which is shaped by race and gender expectations. Positive self-image is even more important for those young adults who, by virtue of being black and female, will have to anticipate barriers throughout adulthood.[5] Parents also teach young adults about gender-appropriate behavior: being a young man or young woman. One sociologist describes the central role of community and family in the development of adolescent beliefs and behavior:

> The strong, so-called decent family, often with a husband and wife, sometimes a strong-willed single mother helped by close relatives and neighbors, may instill in girls a sense of hope. A girl growing up in such a family, or even living in close proximity to one, may have strong social support. . . . [These families] are also able to share knowledge about negotiating life beyond the confines of the neighborhood.[6]

Family bonds are influential in educating teenagers about sex and providing support for decision making. Within the family, parents' willingness to discuss sexual issues, their religious beliefs, and their own sexuality influence children.[7] Young women who abstain from sex report having frequent conversations with their parents regarding sex.

This climate allowed them to feel comfortable with their sexual choices. Parental involvement seems more likely especially when parents fear that their children are at risk of becoming sexually active and when they have clearly defined expectations for their children's achievements and maturation into adulthood.

Teenagers with sexually liberal parents generally are comfortable with the idea of premarital sex. In conservative families, in which sex and sexuality are not discussed, teenagers are expected to maintain their parents' conservative attitudes. In contrast to a popular perception, teenagers from sexually liberal families are not more likely to engage in premarital sex than their conservative peers. Families that are open about sex and also strongly restrict nonmarital sex raise teenagers who *will* postpone sexual activity while retaining positive views of themselves as women.

Young adults should learn about sex and contraception from either a parent or a respected adult role model.[8] Teenagers feel comfortable speaking about these sensitive issues with people they trust. This information should be accurate and relevant to their experiences. In reality, however, many youth first learn about sex from their peers and from popular culture.[9] In rare instances have parents engaged their children in explicit and accurate discussions focused on sex, contraceptives, and sexuality.[10]

Many young women in New Haven reported discussing scientific (i.e., physiological and biological), psychological, or social aspects of sex and reproduction with their parents or guardians. This outcome was initially surprising, because most evidence indicates that the tenuous nature of some young women's family relationships would result in the infrequency or absence of sex-related discussions. In actuality, "discussions" ranged from a cursory treatment of sex to regular conversations about sexual partners and obtaining contraception. There were distinctions by social class in terms of the way information was communicated with the young women. Although the general content of discussions did not fall into neat categories, the way costs, benefits, and motivations were discussed were somewhat different for young women from low-income families in comparison with middle-class teenagers. Parental roles in providing youth with sex education have to be clearly defined, as many parents may not be as involved in regular information sharing with their children as expected.

The majority of poor girls who spoke about sex with a parent (normally the mother or a female guardian) first did so when they were between eleven and thirteen years old. This coincides with the onset of menarche (menstruation); not surprisingly, these conversations were in anticipation of the girls' first menstrual cycle and did not focus on sexual behavior or hormonal changes. Girls who come from middle-class families reported that their parents began to share information with them when they were relatively young. This ranged from one girl's introduction to "how babies are made" in the second grade (approximately seven years old) to another girl's conversation with her parents about why they were having another child.

Arguing that a causal relationship exists between social class and sexual attitudes is too simplistic a viewpoint. There were working poor and poor young women whose parents started to discuss sex with them when they were in elementary school. Little related to social class accounted for the reason some parents started to teach their daughters about sex while they were prepubescent. Most of these parents, according to the young women's descriptions, had progressive sexual attitudes. They did not encourage their daughters to explore their sexuality through intercourse, but they were more willing to entertain their daughters' questions and to provide detailed responses.

In most cases, conversations became more detailed as the girls got older. Even so, the talks tended to center on concern for "changes," "being grown," and "watching out for boys." For poor girls, sex information was packaged as a basic introduction to menstruation and cautionary tales about predatory boys and uncontrollable hormones:

> My mom—she thinks all boys are dogs. Since they are not good and can't be honest, she told me to keep my period to myself so they wouldn't know I was a woman yet.

> So, Aunt Donna sits me down and explains the bleeding to me. I was scared, you know? I mean it's blood. She made me see that bleeding is about being able to have babies and growing. She said I'd start to liking boys—I didn't tell her I already did—and then I would need to take care.

> I knew about having babies—the how part, I mean—pretty young. About nine. I'd tell my friends all the stuff I knew. . . . The period part, that was a little later, about eleven, I think. Then the protection. "Use something, don't bring home diseases." That's what I heard. That being womanly can be good and bad.

The comments of these three young women—ages seventeen, fifteen, and sixteen, respectively—illustrate the "typical" discussions that occurred between parents/caretakers and their daughters.

Some interesting differences emerged in the ways these young women learned about sex. Parents who maintained clear expectations for their children, and who intended for them to finish high school and then work or attend college, were more likely to emphasize three points: sex could be pleasurable, the risks of sex could be long term if they resulted in pregnancy or an STD, and sex is often confused with love. It is possible that these parents were attempting to address the various influences that could cause their children to engage in early sexual activity. Because the perceived emotional benefits of sex often outweigh the eventual benefits of focusing on education and career, young women need to be well prepared for the range of pressures they might face before the end of adolescence.

Among working-poor and poor families, abstinent messages were also used but were different in scope. In most cases parents emphasized two themes: young men were untrustworthy, and there were too many pregnant girls in the community. As one low-income seventeen-year-old observed:

> I never tell them [parents] anything. Sometimes I feel that they can't understand me because they don't know me. Once my mother told me how scared she becomes each time she sees a pregnant teen on the street. She says that's why my dad is being so overprotective, especially about boys. I'm sure she assumes I know enough to keep myself . . . unpregnant. We never talk.

This teenager has lost count of the number of young men with whom she has had multiple sexual encounters but believes there have been at least seven. Currently, she has sexual contact with two men who are in their midtwenties.

What is most interesting about messages focusing on abstinence is that they do not acknowledge the emotions associated with sex, particularly in adolescence, and they do not directly link the immediate appeal of sex with the possible outcomes (risky or not) of sexual intercourse for the young women. Too few abstinence messages from parents directly address living with the risk of HIV infection. The messages of fear of sex and mistrust of men, though commonly used to decrease sexual curiosity, appeared to increase the sense of mystery concerning sex.

Other mechanisms are possible for teaching children about sex in families. Relationships maintained by parents provide strong models that young women can pattern or emulate. Parents who were married or in committed relationships, parents involved in dating various men, and those who did not date (at least to their daughter's knowledge) are all role models who teach the young women in their family about appropriate and inappropriate behaviors and about limitations. In this way teenagers learn about how to deal with their sexual needs.

One case worker describes her role as an intermediary who is part parent, confidant, and teacher for the many clients who have no strong family structure. Without parents or some adult dictating lifestyle and behavioral expectations, young women are becoming increasingly isolated. Her frustration over her fluctuating presence in some teenagers' lives was echoed by Tonnia:

> My mom works hard, so she don't have time to be with us. When she has a double shift we never see her, and when we do, she's flat tired. I love her and know it's hard, but sometimes I miss her. The boys [younger brothers] do whatever, and have no respect for what she do. I tell them to treat her right, but they too busy with some of these girls to care. My girlfriend Roz says that I have a chance to be better with my little girl, and she's right. I want to see her grow up, to be with her every step. But how can I do that when I need to work, and nobody going to just stay with her for free?

Tonnia raised many relevant challenges faced by young women and, more specifically, young mothers. Even those women with close ties to a parent—typically the mother—may not have the opportunity to develop ties with her and learn what life options will and will not interfere with their futures. Rather, trial and error is the method by which some come to experience how decisions can result in lasting, life-altering outcomes.

The presence of parents in the household, though considered a sign of parental involvement, does not mean there is adequate contact with the children in the household. The discomfort young women felt with discussing their sexual behavior and knowledge reflected their parents' discomfort with the same topics. Erratic conversations about reproductive and sexual issues did not prepare young women for the pressures they face in the social world. Teenagers without adequate family support had a weakened sense of social support and thus became reproductive "innovators" who make up expectations and sexual boundaries on a case-by-case basis.[11]

A family is expected to be the primary source of social and emotional support for its members, especially for young adults and children.[12] Whether composed of "blood" relatives or nonrelations, this socially defined unit is almost exclusively responsible for inculcating members under eighteen with guidelines necessary for survival in the world. These guidelines include ones preparing them for adulthood and the creation of their own families.[13] It is enlightening to also consider the messages teenagers receive regarding pregnancy and early parenthood. As with sex education, many parents expressed conflicting attitudes and expectations about pregnancy and parenthood. Conflicting messages greatly influence the perceptions held by young women. For example, if a parent has not impressed on his or her daughter that pregnancy is unacceptable, she may not think about the possible ramifications of being a young parent. Consequently, if a young woman wants to become pregnant or if she feels ambivalent about it, she may not worry about exposure to HIV; contraception—including condoms—will not be a prerequisite for having sex. Wanting to avoid pregnancy does not guarantee that a young woman will use condoms. She may consider other forms of birth control, ones that do not prevent STD infection. What this means, as I will discuss in chapters 5 and 6, is that in addition to fearing pregnancy, a young woman needs to be educated about other issues before she will minimize her risk of infection.

Parents implicitly and explicitly communicate to their children a range of expectations regarding sexuality and parenting. In Wanda's case, her mother and grandmother had frequently impressed upon her that

> sex can only lead to one thing, and that's trouble. . . . They keep telling me about those good-for-nothing types who want your drawers and not the baby that can come after. Mama Allen [Wanda's grandmother] is so excited about all these girls she thinks have babies . . . she says hard work is the only way to be useful. Another child in the world just means another diaper to change [laughs], and she doesn't want to change no more diapers for a long time.

Wanda has dated her boyfriend, who at twenty-two is five years her senior, for two years. They have been sexually active for most of this time, but Wanda uses a condom because she "isn't ready to change diapers, either."

Young women whose parents or mentors discussed pregnancy outcomes and the social ramifications of these options were more likely to defer pregnancy by either abstaining from sex or using contraception. In these cases, pregnancy was not just one of many life changes available to young women. They were exposed to "traditional" middle-class social values; pregnancy represented risk, negative life outcomes, and a shift in social status *for the worst*, as these comments illustrate:

> It's very simple. If I have a baby, I get to pack my things and leave. My parents would never let me get pregnant and have a baby under their roof. It disrespects their name and everything. As long as I'm in their house, I live by their rules.

Someday I want a few children, but not now. I couldn't handle them because I'm too young. I have a cousin who'd gotten herself into trouble a few years ago. I remember folks talking badly about what she did. She opened her legs and things. I felt bad for her because she had it so hard. Her mother helped her out but didn't like it. Imagine going to Thanksgiving or Christmas and having people smiling and still talking about you?

I was watching TV with my friend. The stories were on, I guess *All My Children*. I think Dixie was pregnant by Adam. You know how he is. . . . When she [respondent's mother] saw her looking like she did Mom went off. About how no young lady should be shacked up with any old man, even a rich one.

In comparison with these middle-class teens, Leslie, whose parents were working poor, did not have a clear sense of what her family expected or would tolerate. Life expectations had not been clearly identified while she was growing up.

You know, my grandmom and aunt had theirs kinda young. My mom had us right after she got married. One after another. That's not my thing, though. I know she had a hard time with us, and Grandma too. . . . She probably would be okay if I got pregnant, if I could handle it. I think she knows about me and Roy [Leslie's boyfriend], but she deals with it. She just smiles at us, sometimes.

Messages young women receive from their parents are even more ambiguous than this. In Leslie's case, knowing about her mother's reproductive history has apparently made her more cautious about motherhood, even though she rarely discussed the specifics with her mother.

In other situations, either parents were completely uncommunicative or they gave off contradictory messages. Contradictions sometimes arose in what each of the parents said to the young woman. Mothers generally represented a potential source of information, while fathers often made comments that provided a different view of what was expected from the daughter. For example, Dara's father routinely made disparaging comments about young men in the community who had expressed interest in her:

Daddy's way overdone. You know, last week we were in the mall and Paul came by and said, "What's up?" and Dad went off, saying that he was disrespectful in how he was acting. Now daddy's got my interest in mind, but why's he gotta do that? [H]e doesn't think that boys around here . . . are worth my time at all.

Her mother, however, "wants me to get myself together and marry somebody!! She says when I turn eighteen I got to go and make my own way. I just think she's wanting my room for a den or something!"

Message content might contradict with how parents responded to others' behavior. Some parents and relatives behaved in ways that encouraged their children to seriously consider pregnancy as an option. Julianna talked about a shopping trip she took with an aunt:

> In Macy's on the second floor is where the kids' clothes are. We walked by it and A'Drienne took one look at a little bitty dress and told me "couldn't you see a baby in this? What do you think?" I said no way, and we looked around. We kept finding outfits that would be nice for babies. I think Baby Gap is better, though . . . I know exactly how my child would dress—he'd always be really neat.

While A'Drienne did not explicitly tell Julianna that pregnancy was acceptable, she did encourage her to imagine what being a mother was like without offering any rejoinders on the need to wait until Julianna was older.

By emphasizing the importance of school, employment, and delayed parenting, adult role models can affect adolescents' and children's future actions. A mother has a special role because she

> is in a position to impress upon her daughter the importance of education, and is able to take a more active role in her daughter's academic process. . . . [T]he more highly educated a mother is, the less authoritarian in her childrearing practices, and her children have higher educational goals than the children of mothers with less education. These mothers may act as positive role models, inspiring their daughters to strive for academic success.[14]

However, those parents who are considered excessively restrictive or permissive face the risk of raising children who reject their norms in favor of opposite ones. What this discussion indicates is that there is a myriad of other influences on the attitudes, beliefs and behaviors of young adults.

The Sisterhood: Girlfriends and Peers

Adolescent behavior, sexual and otherwise, is supposed to be affected by peer pressure and young people's search for identity through group membership and group acceptance. As a member of a particular group or subculture—often referred to as a reference group within social psychology literature—an individual is expected to abide by the

values, codes of behavior, and morals defined by the collective. Ultimately, identity is affected by one's peer group: "[s]elf and social evaluation can come about in one of two ways. In the first, the individual
accepts the evaluations expressed by others and applies them to [her]-
self . . . The second way in which self (or social) evaluation can come
about is through a process of comparison with others."[15] A young
woman identifies with a social group and assumes the characteristics
associated with this group; she develops a sense of self by comparing
herself with others in the social world.

Concern for the impact of peer pressure on adolescent behavior is a
logical outgrowth of this school of thought. Peer groups are one source
of socialization, along with family, school, religious institutions, and
so on. The way teenagers teach each other about sex and AIDS would
affect how they will subsequently behave. If they associate with people
who engage in high-risk activities, then logically they, too, would be
inclined to do the same.[16] In measuring the relative importance of peer
groups (or sexual/romantic partners) on sexual activity, some studies
have surveyed how teenagers perceive themselves and how they feel
others see them as a way to estimate how responsive they are to peer
pressure.[17] Young adults who seek group acceptance and approval are
more willing to behave in ways that they think reflect their peers' behaviors. They are also more likely to reject behaviors that are identified
with unpopular groups.[18]

Teenagers spend more social time with peers than with their adult
relatives and parents. Do they also spend more time talking about sex
and sexual behavior with their peers? More specifically, how do they
use friends as sources of knowledge? As reference group theory suggests, a young woman's primary social cohort is where she refines her
expectations, attitudes, and beliefs concerning a range of issues. Few
of the teenagers, when asked, admitted to maintaining regular discussions with their friends about sex. This is not to say that these discussions never happened. Many implied that in general they depended
on their girlfriends for support, advice, and information regarding sex.
Frequent conversations about sex were not necessary. Merely knowing
that their friends were sympathetic was enough. Eva remembers one
of her first "lessons" on sex, from her best friend in the fourth grade:

> Janet told me that she had saw some boy's thing up close, by mistake. He
> was peeing and left the door open. After he was done, he turned and she
> got a look. She told me it looked real nasty and all that. . . . She says that
> poking a penis in all sorts of places can get you sick or make you get
> pregnant. We still wanted to see another one up really close.

Peers' role in introducing each other to issues of sexual identity was extremely important. Openness about sex took the form of stories such as the one related by Eva. Sharing stories about people, particularly celebrities, was another tool used to learn about sex.

The topic of sex often was raised during conversations about friends and peers. Gossip and speculation about sexual availability, parties, who was dating whom, and the lives of celebrities offered opportunities for informal sex education. During one conversation, two friends embarked on a lively discussion about one young woman's sexual tastes.

> **Doreen:** I'm sorry, but that girl is just a freak! I heard about some of the shit she has gotten into.
>
> **Ruth:** Back in the day, [Maureen] was normal. But she thinks she has to get into all sorts of things to keep a man. There isn't any man worth doing that with. I mean, first of all, she's pullin' trains [when a woman has sex with a series of men in a brief period of time—often within a few hours, and sometimes against her will] and just to do that! You couldn't pay me to do that.
>
> **Doreen:** Well, I heard that last week she was at [a local club] and that she just dogged Anthony by rubbing up against anyone who'd have her. No pride. Now so many guys know about her and what she'll do that they don't give the rest of us the kind of respect we deserve!

They were referring to the rumor that a young woman willingly engaged in, and often initiated, oral sex. From their conversation, it became apparent that oral sex was taboo and that one's reputation was dependent upon the kinds of sex you enjoyed. Although this conversation was not intended to educate anyone, both young women were reinforcing and validating their sexual value systems.

Rarely did the young women describe situations in which they explicitly requested information from a friend or explained something concerning sexual activity to others. Young women kept references to their own sexual activity to themselves, but they were willing to discuss pregnancy scares, menstruation, and contraception. Euphemisms were used in reference to menstruation. It was called everything from "the curse" and "my thing" to "a guest," "my visitor," and "it." There appeared to be a great deal of embarrassment associated with discussions of the basics of reproduction and bodily changes. Young women were much more comfortable talking about sex in the abstract and about their platonic relationships with friends.

Throughout my interviews, young women frequently referred to the importance of having friends to turn to in times of emotional difficulty. Niobe Way's study of teenage boys and girls in New York City reinforces the importance of peer support but with a qualification.[19] Youth reported feeling cautious about developing and maintaining friendships. They were uncomfortable disclosing private information. Older teenagers were especially protective but were also very nostalgic about past friendships. This was particularly true of teenage girls. The vast majority would approach a girlfriend with a personal problem before going to a parent or relative (the only notable exception was sisters close in age to the young women). In fact, if a friend was not available, most stated that they would simply keep their concerns to themselves and, as one said, "try to figure out what to do without causing a commotion or worrying family."

Even though sexually active teenage girls knew that many of their peers were active (or that rumors attested to that fact), they rarely perceived themselves as part of a peer community in which they were expected and encouraged to have sex. At the same time, seeing other girls reap the imagined benefits of sexual activity was not lost on them. Thus, the question of peer pressure, and how it is manifested, emerges.[20] Do young women pursue sex because their friends and peers do so? Is this because the benefits of sexual activity outweigh the costs (in the opinion of their social contacts—their "points of reference")? Although this project did not allow for the subtle distinctions at play in these questions, many of the girls I encountered provided some potential points of departure. I specifically asked some teenage mothers about their pregnancies being the result of peer pressure. At one point, we talked about others' influencing their sexual activity:

Denise: I think it's stupid to do it 'cause of someone. Don't these girls have sense? You know the saying about jumping off of a bridge. I mean be serious. Umm . . . does someone come up to you with a gun and demand that you have sex? Girls do it because they want to and 'cause no one can stop them.

Robin: Maybe if you start getting into sex real young, maybe before fourteen, it's through pressure. Yeah, probably the guy, I'd think. I have never heard about a girl pressuring someone to have sex.

RTW: If you think of it as less obvious. Could a friend convince you to consider doing something because they've done something like it?

Robin: Are you thinking, like what?

RTW: Like sex. You know, the whole thing.

Denise: Hell, not with me. Girls, I mean, women . . . well, you know?

We don't get fooled easily. Sometimes maybe I'd think about
something if a friend had said something, but no.
Robin: But isn't that it?
Denise: What's it?
Robin: Doing a thing 'cause a friend does it.
Denise: And you've never been there too?

Of interest in this exchange is the claim that they were not subject to
peer pressure. Perhaps peer pressure, as opposed to role modeling, is
effective only if the young women are aware that their peers have set
expectations for them.

An individual models her behavior in accordance with the parameters set by the group with which she most closely identifies. Belonging
to a group, being recognized as someone others like and appreciate, is
especially important for teenagers and young adults. One's perception
of herself as a woman is influenced in part by friends. The more a
young woman depends on others for a positive view of herself, the
more likely it is that she will change in response to the expectations of
other teenagers. Self-image (concerning sexuality) and esteem influence how susceptible a young woman will be to peer pressure.

Conceptually, peer pressure has become a catchall phrase used to
explain the negative influences of "socially undesirable" youth on
"good" teenagers.[21] It is being used to explain why young adults engage in socially unacceptable behavior. Of equal concern is the presence and influence of role models in the lives of young adults. Although they can affect a teenager either positively or negatively, in
terms of sexual activity and pregnancy, some argue that role models
are the antidote for teenagers' problematic behavior.[22]

There has been some interest in the existence of racial differences in
susceptibility to peer pressure. In comparing white and black teenagers, two researchers[23] concluded that among tenth graders in high
schools where peers are not critical of out of wedlock births, white
teenage females are more likely than black teenagers to consider becoming pregnant and having the child. This remained true when background variables were controlled for. However, according to Dore and
Dumois (1990), white teenagers who are not concerned with peer approval are more likely to make reproductive decisions based on what
they want rather than on what their peers expect.[24] Maintaining high
esteem is not dependent on peer approval. But black teens whose esteem is affected by peers are more likely to behave in ways that will
gain the approval of others. Contradictory findings exist concerning
racial-ethnic differences in susceptibility to intraracial peer pressure.

Many black teenage females were very aware of their sexuality and were sometimes self-conscious. Self-consciousness did not always translate into excessive sensitivity to others' opinions and their need to seek the approval of others. The young black women in this project were not particularly swayed to have sex merely because their friends had done so. However, more were likely to report that they had a child, or were considering pregnancy, because of a friend. Young women were not responsive to negative messages from friends; being told not to do something had little influence on what they would do. However, being encouraged to behave in a certain way often resulted in a young woman acting on these impulses. For example, most teenagers became pregnant because they did not care about the threat of negative social sanctions from peers or others. A lack of concern over social sanction reflects the ambiguous boundaries set by older relatives and parents regarding appropriate and inappropriate life choices. Gerry, age seventeen, is pregnant with her second child. She knows that one of her friends was upset when informed of the pregnancy; however, she was not concerned because

> this baby is going to be loved anyway. Charlene will come around—she always does. I am happy about this one, because I am older and can be a better mother. My first one I had at fifteen. I was a baby too. . . . Charlene is my best and closest girlfriend so I wish she'd be happy for me, but it's going to happen anyway. She'll make a good godmother.

Explicit disapproval was, as Gerry explained, disappointing but after the fact. Teenagers were generally less affected by negative peer sanctions of pregnancy whether these were expressed before or after a pregnancy occurred.

I found that young women, although not easily influenced by peer pressure, are influenced by implicitly defined behavioral norms.[25] In a community where a large number of teenagers are pregnant, the underlying negative sanctions associated with single parenthood are minimized.[26] If a young woman's primary social support lies with other teenage mothers and pregnant teens, then pregnancy becomes a viable option. "I've already seen what having a baby is about," said Evelyn. "Some of the girls on my block have kids, so I know I could handle a baby." Young women do not have to express in concrete terms that they are expected to conceive; observing this as a social norm is sufficient. Peer pressure becomes a factor only if she will be socially disadvantaged by not becoming pregnant.

Though sensitive to how others responded to their behaviors, the sexually active teenagers were less concerned than abstinent teens about others' assessments of their behavior. A few conflicting elements are at work. First, young women with an extensive sexual history became active in order to attain adult status. Once they felt this was achieved, they generally expressed satisfaction with themselves. It would not be inconsistent, though, for surveys to indicate that they score high on self-image while scoring low on measurement of comfort with their sexuality.[27] Such conflicting feelings are reflected when they report regret over the timing of their initial sexual activity while claiming to be satisfied with having initiated sex at a young age.

Teenagers who were most likely to be affected by peer pressure were ones who feared a loss of social status. These were young women who avoided pregnancy in order to retain the approval of their friends. Though they did not explicitly discuss how peer pressure became a gatekeeper of behavior, many did realize that their public persona could be damaged by pregnancy:

> I can't see myself pregnant, let alone with a little baby. You know, I see those girls in school and on the street, and I wonder what they are thinking and feeling. . . . I mean, I would kill my best friend if she ever did that.

> The whole "good girl" and "bad girl" thing is unfair, but that's life. Like if you lay down with dogs, you get fleas. I'm not saying these girls are dogs or anything, just that people look at you funny. Immediately you're seen for what's between your legs, not what's in your head. Everyone says that, but it is true.

Distancing themselves from pregnant teenagers was one mechanism used by those young women who defined pregnancy as a downward shift in status. Karen drew a comparison between pregnant teenagers and herself in a similar way:

> I see girls, some old friends, who have one, two, or more kids. What are they doing to themselves? Obviously raising kids gets in the way of school. Especially in the way of college. They just don't care, and they are irresponsible. I have no interest in living like that. They seem happy, but how can they be when they give up life as a teenager?

Children and teenagers define themselves through membership in a peer group. Continued membership in this group is determined by their ability to conform to the values and norms associated with the group. At the same time, however, one's membership in a group affords her the opportunity to redefine these value systems. There is a problem with claiming that peer pressure is to blame for sexual behavior. Making this argument requires presuming that teenagers are passive receptacles into whom others merely project their own wishes. A young woman is not merely a passive member in the social collective, one who reacts to what is expected of her. She is constantly refining her family-based value system and the one defined by peers and larger social networks into her own personal system.

A young woman susceptible to peer pressure would tend to alter her attitudes and actions in response to her perceptions of peers' expectations because of her need to assume and maintain a particular status within a peer group and her need to attain external validation. Perceived expectations, the need for status attainment, and even participation in peer groups fluctuate in response to broader social phenomena. Societal concern over the relationship between peer pressure and teenage pregnancy is on some level an expression of concern over social values shifting in response to changing institutional structures.[28]

The impetus behind teenage pregnancy, whether planned or not, is partly determined by the presence of peers who are either pregnant or who would be supportive of others' pregnancies. "My girlfriend and me wanted to have our babies at the same time," said Evelyn, a fifteen-year-old first-time parent, "that way we could share everything together. . . . [I] have always known I would get someone to make me pregnant because it seems like fun. Why not? I can love her as good as these other girls can." While it would be a natural assumption to label this peer pressure, such an observation would only address one part of the issue.

Peer group beliefs are developed in the context of shifting social mores. For example, pregnancy and parenthood are traditionally adult experiences. For teenagers who wish to hasten their entry into adulthood, parenthood becomes one feasible means of doing so. While experiencing pressure from friends to behave as adults, these teenagers are also responding to the social definition of what adulthood and maturity mean—namely, parenthood. In considering what sex, pregnancy, parenthood, and childbirth represent to teenagers, we need also to consider how these are valued in a wider social framework.

Although relationships with family and friends are greatly influential in the emotional and social development of young women, an additional element is influential as well—social class. Whenever a social scientist, political, policy maker, educator, or counselor addresses sexual behavior among teenagers, the question of class background is raised. As some of the studies mentioned make clear, social class seems to have a place in this discussion. Where one grows up, the people she encounters, and the resources at her disposal are all affected to some extent by economic factors. At times these factors are tangible, as in the amount of food she will have on the table, the kinds of clothes she wears, or the kinds of neighborhoods in which her family can or cannot live. But what is also of interest and importance are the less tangible elements of social class. Privilege and opportunity bring with them the promise of a certain kind of future and the presumption of a particular kind of social status denied many low-income teenagers. This basic reality continually shapes whom young women encounter, how they relate to others, and what decisions they make regarding their own lives.

Learning to Be Women

Young women learn so many things from those around them. It is important to recognize that this learning process occurs even when people are not actively involved in it; learning about becoming a woman, entering adulthood, and all that this entails can occur both actively and passively. So what exactly do young women learn from others that affects sexuality and sexual behavior? They learn what symbolizes adulthood, what to expect in relationships and friendships, whether they should trust other people, the value to be placed about sex, and potentially unanticipated outcomes of sexual behavior: pregnancy and HIV infection.

Being a woman, growing into adulthood, is of utmost importance to most teenage girls. They learn that they can attain these goals a number of possible ways: by achieving academic and occupational/financial success, by having children, by entering into a relationship with an older man, and, in some cases, by having sex on a regular basis. Watching adult women in their families and communities has a lasting impression on which avenue a teenager will choose. Conversations in which adult role models talk about women in the community are as influential as more direct messages. Fathers or other adult males certainly influence this process of discovery by showing young women how they should or may be treated by men. Here again, what occurs within the home can leave lifelong imprints, whether negative or positive.

Friendships are the site of a different sort of learning process. One can experiment with different behaviors, talk about dreams and expectations, share information as well as seek it from peers. As young women mature, naturally the nature and function of their friendships change. Some friends are identified as more trustworthy, as the ones most likely to provide support regardless of the circumstances. Watching how others behave and seeing the effects of their behavior provide a range of messages for a young woman. The risk of losing face in public, and possibly being embarrassed, causes many teenagers to be very cautious about what they share with whom. Ultimately, though, the experimentation and personality transformations that are endemic to adolescence are facilitated by friendships.

4

Building Relationships: Love, Dating, and Romance

At the heart of the mystery concerning teenagers and sexually transmitted diseases is the nature of intimate relationships and love. Although some teenagers do not pursue or want to be involved in a long-term relationship during high school, the majority seem to place a great deal of emphasis on looking for, maintaining, and ending romantic relationships. The importance of intimacy, the ways young men and women court each other, and the nature and substance of relationships are all issues of concern here for a number of reasons. First, there may be a connection between the importance placed on dating and a young woman's willingness to participate in high risk sexual behaviors with a man. Second, the way teenagers perceive or define normal relationships may provide insight into their ability to communicate with a partner their own concerns regarding AIDS and HIV. Understanding the roles sex and sexuality play in their lives also requires considering the nature of teenage relationships. Finally, there is much we do not know about the effects of wider societal factors on the maintenance of relationships. Clarifying all of these unknowns would enable us to address risk taking among teenagers much more effectively than we currently do.

Social scientists have attempted to isolate the factors most closely related to the initiation of sexual intercourse and the extent to which teenagers risk (unknowingly or consciously) contracting STDs. One scholar has identified eleven factors that appear to influence a young adult's decision to have sex.[1] Six of these are institutional or environmental factors; they concern access to health care, educational background, the nature of social relationships a woman has, employment levels in her community and family, and the general economic conditions she faces. The remaining five factors are cultural or values oriented: attitudes and beliefs concerning marriage, child bearing, contraception, abortion, and sex. This all-inclusive list illustrates that sexual behavior and intimate relations are affected by personal, lifestyle, and societal/structural factors.

Unfortunately, teenagers' sexuality and ideas regarding intimacy still remain among the most understudied issues in sociology,[2] partly because it is so difficult to convince teenagers to talk about their most personal and intimate relationships and partly because of necessary restrictions on the explicitness of conversations researchers can have with teenagers. A great deal of information concerns whether teenagers are sexually active, the frequency of this activity, as well as the numbers of young women who regularly date. What are less studied are what teenagers think about sex and how they behave in relationships with young men.

Adolescence is a period of self-discovery and experimentation. Studying the stages through which a young woman's identity and relationships with men evolve can contribute to our understanding of her sexual behavior and her willingness or unwillingness to take sexual risks. Do young adults actually court each other anymore? Where and how do they initiate relationships? We need to consider systematically how they define romance and what happens when they fall in love. To what extent do gender and sex roles shape relationships? Answering all of these questions necessitates looking at the social environment in which these issues gain importance.

The world in which we live appears to be more complicated and unpredictable. Within popular discourse are social scientists and cultural essayists who either bemoan or celebrate the changes in gender and sex roles within the United States. Women are delaying marriage because of educational and career opportunities, and many do not have children until in their late thirties or forties. The divorce rate hovers somewhere between 50 and 60 percent. More women are assuming competitive jobs with high levels of responsibility. Additionally, women are making inroads in traditionally male occupations. Naturally all of these changes have influenced the way men and women interact.

Children and teenagers are maturing in the midst of these rapid and sometimes short-lived changes. Messages concerning gender-appropriate behavior in mixed-sex environments remain conflictual and confusing. Much of the dialogue about the way men and women relate has trickled down to children and teenagers. For example, magazine surveys indicate that teenagers are increasingly aware of unwanted sexual advances and harassment. At least 70 percent of girls between thirteen and seventeen recently surveyed by *Seventeen* magazine reported having experienced unwanted comments, touching, fondling, or more invasive acts while at school. Just a few years ago, many of these same behaviors would have not warranted as much concern among young women. In 1996, a few cases of sexual harassment gained public attention. These cases are relevant to the question of gender and relationships because they illustrate how erratic gender role expectations have become. In New York City, a child in kindergarten was suspended for having kissed a girl. A few weeks later the same thing happened to a young boy in another state. Both of these situations raised the issue of the unstable and erratic imposition of gender boundaries. What kinds of physicality are allowable and in what situations? If one comments on a woman's appearance, is that flattery or sexual aggression? Because adults remain unclear about such questions, then shouldn't teenagers feel the same?

Many popular courtship and relationship books are on the market, including *Men Are from Mars, Women Are from Venus* and one of the latest additions to the discourse, *The Rules*. Books dealing with time-honored questions about the "battle of the sexes" have increased in popularity at least in part because male and female social and sexual roles are less restrictive and bounded. Women in particular have more freedom and flexibility to behave in ways previously denied them. The confusion that authors of relationship self-help books seek to resolve is the same confusion experienced by young women. As they face contradictory expectations, and deal with young men and friends, teenage girls encounter many questions and few solutions.

Teenage Romance: Where Is the Research?

Young women learn about relationships from different kinds of sources. Expectations they maintain for their relationship are such an important part of sexual behavior and contraceptive decision making. It is therefore troubling to note that so few studies of HIV, AIDS, teen pregnancy, or sexuality deal comprehensively or exclusively with teenage relationships. Some of the most noteworthy sociological works on the nature of gender identity and adolescent sexuality completely overlook an instrumental element of the story: how relationships develop.[3] Considering that on some level sexuality is associated with intimate relationships, why do studies of dating during adolescence focus primarily on trends in sexual intercourse? What such an assumption does is dismiss and minimize the obvious importance placed on the process leading to the development of a relationship. Not all teenagers' romantic relationships solely concern sexual intercourse. It is in fact dangerous to claim that teenagers are purely driven by hormones and instinct and that all of their intimate sexual relations are "puppy love." All too often people assume that because teenagers are young and less experienced than adults, they do not or cannot experience the kinds of emotional upheaval adults encounter in their own intimate relationships.

People often maintain contradictory views about gender roles throughout the course of their lives. They start addressing these contradictions while very young and continue to "try on" various identities by rehearsing different roles in each relationship. As societal definitions change, so does the gender role-play within relationships. Gender roles, our cultural definitions of appropriate behavior for men and women, certainly are associated with the development of relationships. What happens in a relationship is a microcosm of wider societal gender norms. All the gender-related conflict and contradiction can be intensified in such an intimate setting.

We are socialized to behave according to a set of expectations based on characteristics such as race, age, and gender. As there are behaviors deemed appropriate and inappropriate for members of a particular age group, there are also clearly defined gender expectations we start to learn as infants. We watched how adults interact with each other: the way they maintain physical contact, use their voices, dress, and so on. As children we were taught by family, teachers, friends, and the media to engage in behaviors acceptable and appropriate for our sex. Athletic girls become "tomboys," and quiet boys become "sissies." Children experiment with gender roles in games such as "playing house." Everywhere they turn children confront a multitude of rules that appear to be simultaneously predictable and changeable.[4] It seems obvious, then, that teenagers, especially younger ones, will continue to play out and experiment with all of these gender expectations in their own relationships—including sexual ones.

> Young adolescents' sexual behaviors both influence and are influenced by adolescents' conceptions of masculinity and femininity. . . . Although conceptions of gender roles have changed in the recent past, males appear to be more traditional than females. . . . Gender-role norms regarding power in male-female relationships appear to be related to adolescents' developing sexual conduct.[5]

The playing out of such gender identities and roles will influence the resolution of questions concerning sexual activity and contraception use.

Although young women in the late twentieth century are the product of a feminist sensibility, they are also aware of traditional gender norms and at some point begin to enact elements of these norms. Using what has been called sexual scripts, they play out expected female roles with young men. In his study of a black neighborhood, one sociologist observed, "The girls have a dream, the boys a desire. The girls dream of being carried off by a Prince Charming who will love them, provide for them, and give them a family. The boys often desire sex without commitment, or babies without responsibility for them."[6] Although young adults may not be as self-aware of their intentions as Elijah Anderson (1990) implies, what appears true is that the continuing persuasiveness of traditional gender norms have influenced young black women's relationship expectations.

Studies of gender norms within various social economic levels have indicated that marked social class differences exist in terms of gender-appropriate behavior.[7] Regardless of race, some have noted that within low-income families and communities are contradictory expectations of women. On the one hand, women are expected to participate in maintaining the household by working, but at the same time, their intimate interactions assume stereotypically traditional behavior. Given that the popular culture in the United States offers these contradictory gender images for mass consumption, it may not be so far-fetched that some young adults get the message: "Girls realize very early that one of the ways to achieve the status of a woman is to learn the more complex game that is involved in interpersonal male-female relationships."[8] Poor and working-class girls face a double jeopardy of sorts. They are aware of the pressure to conform to stereotypically feminine activity. They are also aware that contemporary female norms allow for independence and self-sufficiency in the public sphere. However, they have few opportunities to realize this contemporary expectation.

Young women from low-income families manage these dichotomous gender expectations by behaving in traditional ways around their boyfriends. A theoretical perspective may shed some light on what low-income teenagers experience. Life course theorists claim that a range of structural factors (such as economics) affect the speed with which teenagers mature.[9] Poor communities tend to operate like preindustrial and early industrial societies. The residents face high mortality rates, extreme economic stress, and social-political isolation from other communities. Children are expected to marry or pair off while young and to assume adult responsibilities, because many presume that they will not live as long as residents in more economically and socially stable communities. In a sense, the youth experience a brief adolescence and may not face extreme sanction for engaging in typically adult behavior.

Activities associated with adulthood are unavailable to low-income teenagers because of educational and occupational barriers. If they cannot attain certain socially valued goals such as a college education, upwardly mobile work, and marriage, then the only available option is to improvise some approximation of adult behavior.[10] What is an option is to appear *womanly* in their intimate relationships. The young black women in this book frequently explained that their educational and financial accomplishment was important to a relative or mentor. However, those who had little faith in their ability to attain this component of contemporary black womanhood might find themselves relying on stereotypical gender behavior. Although many expressed strongly feminist rhetoric such as the importance of egalitarian gender roles in relationships and the benefits of remaining financially independent of men, they often in the same breath expressed strongly traditional expectations of young men's romantic behavior and described situations in which they were passive participants in relationships with their partners. One way to successfully maintain a boyfriend is by embodying traditional gender scripts of womanhood.

Most studies have concluded that young women who adhere to traditional views of masculine and feminine behavior tend to be more willing to give in to their male partners' needs and wishes.[11] Maintaining traditional gender norms within a relationship means that the ways the partners interact with each other, and what they expect, will reflect more normative kinds of gender roles for men and women: women caretake and cooperate, and men take charge and establish relationship rules. As far as sexual interactions are concerned, if the boyfriend wishes to engage in unprotected or other forms of risky sex and the young woman defers to her traditional role, then the young woman is making a potentially dangerous choice concerning HIV infection. For example, "for a woman to insist on condoms with a reluctant male partner requires discussion at each sexual encounter, often demanding that a woman have influence over a man in a setting that is highly emotionally charged and fraught with social meaning."[12] Conversely, when teenage girls maintain egalitarian sex roles in their relationships, they are more likely to communicate about contraception and about their needs with their partners.[13]

Young women are often socialized into assuming stereotypically dependent or nonassertive gender roles in another way. In "Sexuality, Schooling and Adolescent Females: The Missing Discourse of Desire," Michelle Fine (1988) observes that many school-supported sex education programs use an approach in which

[t]he language, as well as the questions asked and not asked, represents females as the actual and potential victims of male desire. In exercises, role plays, and class discussions, girls practice resistance to trite lines, unwanted hands, opened buttons, and the surrender of other "bases" they are not prepared to yield. The discussions of violence and victimization both portray males as potential predators and females as victims.[14]

Fine argues that all too often young women are taught to be victims. They are taught to expect that they must assume passive roles around men and to expect sexual aggression from men. Sexual exploitation becomes an anticipated reality in relationships.

Making such a claim does not mean we should ignore the reality of sexual exploitation of young women. In fact, the question of exploitation and abuse is a relevant and timely one, particularly for teenagers involved with older adult men.[15] In fact, a series of studies have identified that a history of abuse and sexual exploitation—whether at the hands of a parent, relative, or boyfriend—greatly affects a woman's ability to accurately assess and protect herself from risk.[16] For example, victims of sexual abuse are likely to initiate sexual relationships at a young age and to engage in very high-risk sexual activities (particularly multiple sexual partners). Again, a young woman in an exploitative romantic relationship may behave out of fear and intimidation rather than assert herself.

A handful of researchers have begun to allude to the importance of investigating teenagers' relationships. In studying sexuality, sexual activity, and contraception, they have recognized the powerful influence intimate sexual and emotional relationships may have on a child's or young adult's attitudes, beliefs, and behavior. In a few instances authors provide very comprehensive views of the romantic lives of teenage girls[17] and women[18] and how these relationships actually determine the extent of sexual risk taking.

"Getting" a Man

Caryn and her friend James have been together for about eighteen months. She describes him as being "fine, but not too fine. If he were any cuter he might begin looking at too many of the ladies." Having been together for over a year marks their relationship as relatively serious. Some of Caryn's friends consider her an authority on the subject of relationships and consult her for dating advice. Because of this esteemed social position, she was more self-aware and conversant about the "how-to's" of dating. In relating how she and James first met, it was apparent that group contact was an important part of the process:

> At the park they were playing hoops, and we went to hang and watch them. Sherese was checking this guy out—I think it was Rodney. I saw James and kinda noticed him because he could play really good. I know he saw me watching and he started showing off, so of course he started messing up! You know—trying to act cute.

The characterization of courtship as a cat and mouse game was particularly true in Caryn's case. Once she knew that she had been noticed, she started "actively" to ignore him in public group encounters. Although the need to protect the ego and save face is at least partly the motive, it seems as if this was also an element of a time-honored ritual. Each party wants to feel secure before making a noticeable and personal commitment to a relationship.

Though many studies of black sexual activity conclude that intercourse occurs early in the romantic relationship,[19] they often do not recognize that the period of courtship leading to committed relationships might be extensive. What this indicates is that though the window of time between first dating and having sex may be brief, on occasion teenagers may in fact be much more deliberative about their partner selection than expected. Without generalizing too extensively, we might say that many young women followed closely a system of courtship.

Nothing has changed over the decades of courtship among men and women. Physical appearance is still what attracts many young adults to each other. How a man looks, what he wears, and how he carries himself are interpreted as indicators of a range of character traits. Keeping himself up obviously indicates that a young man cares about how he looks but also that he probably cares about what his girlfriend wears. Apart from status, wearing the correct labels signifies that he is willing to spend some of his money. Observation and "precourtship" occur at school as well as during trips to and from school and in shopping malls. Various social interactions and exchanges take place outside school. Public spaces allow for people to project, and absorb, visual images that communicate volumes about their personality.

In public settings groups of teenagers can observe and interact with each other with a minimum of risk and a maximum of assertiveness. Three main shopping malls are in close proximity to New Haven. After school and on weekends high-volume activity occurs throughout these centers. Food courts are especially popular sites. In these areas young men and women can watch each other and comment on what they see while appearing to be completely engrossed in a different activity—finding something to eat. Watching this deceptively simple interaction, much becomes apparent. Some of the "rules of the game" involve two groups contacting each other before couples pair off. Often the young women initiate contact with young men nonverbally, which leads to conversing and possibly pairing off, but rarely anything more.

What is especially interesting is that on weekends young women prepare for a trip to the mall as if they were going to a party. Even those dressed very casually often took great pains to achieve their look. I saw two young women—best friends—in many public settings where they were dressed identically. Their uniform of choice included baggy jeans, hiking boots, sweatshirts featuring the DKNY, Nike, or Ralph Lauren/Polo logo, thick braids, and long manicured nails.

RTW: I noticed that the two of you often dress alike.
JV: Yeah, it's fun. People notice.
RTW: So how do you decide what to wear?
JV: I don't know. We just talk about it and then make sure we've got the same thing.
RTW: Then you shop together too?
JV: Well, of course! We'll go pick up gear on weekends, for parties and school. That usual thing. . . . My mother is always telling me that my drag looks dumb because we dress the same, but this lets folks know how tight we two are. We're a package deal.

Whenever Jenette and her friend went shopping, they made sure to dress similarly if not identically. She claimed that they had been approached by young men who liked their "twin style." Though dressing alike reflected that they took some effort to dress a certain way, remaining casual indicated that they were not dressing to impress anyone, even men. In reality, though, image and presentation of public self is usually a prime motivation. Appearing sexually appealing to men is also of great concern during adolescence. Being able to get someone's attention and impressing him enough for him to approach you is a validation of womanliness. Those who wear sexually revealing clothes are quite aware of the response they will get. "I like it when they call to me. It makes me feel sexy when they slow down in their cars or maybe honk," explains one. According to another teenager, "I feel powerful when putting on those things. You know, I could have any man I want. It lets them know that I'm definitely *not* playing around. I know what I want." So young women are as aware of the importance of their looks as they are concerned about the appearance of the young men they meet.

Young women spend energy discussing and evaluating various young men in abstract terms. Admitting personal interest is something reserved for the closest friend. Peer support is particularly important before a girl would make any overtures toward a male. Frequent conversations speculating on availability, character, build, dress, and financial stability take place before a girl admitted her interest. Even then, her admission could be very casual and depersonalized. In a conversation overheard before an after-school program, one girl nonchalantly expressed her interest in a well-liked boy who also participated in the program.[20]

Girl 1: He's seriously fine. I mean, foooine!
Girl 2: He's all right.
Girl 3: What's with all right? He IS cute. I heard he broke up with————.
Girl 1: For real? You lie. She wouldn't let him go unless she was beat down by somebody.
Girl 3: Well, that's what I heard.
Girl 2: So he's looking, right?
Girl 1: You know he is. He won't waste any time hooking with someone new.
Girl 2: Uh-huh.
Girl 3: Go on, girlfriend. You know what you need to do. [laughter]
Girl 2: Like I said. I think he's okay.

During a break that afternoon, these three young women were engaged in heated conversation when "Girl 2" quickly walked over to a table near the object of their previous conversation. Within a few minutes he sat next to her and they began to talk. Meanwhile, her two girlfriends watched intently and giggled.

Parties offer another opportunity for young men and women to meet. These settings are formally recognized as sites where relationships may develop. For some, house parties provide the chance for quick sexual encounters with men who were not "relationship material." For most, though, sexual contact is neither the sole nor the primary purpose of a party. Instead, it enables young women to observe a large number of men in a brief period of time. Some still perceive parties as meat markets where they are on display and have a short period of time in which to attract a potential male partner. Meeting a prospective date or boyfriend at a friend's house provides yet another safe space in which to "check someone out" without having committed to an actual date. It is evident that image management and self-protection are definitely issues for most teenagers—whether male or female. They wish to develop intimate connections with each other but fear rejection and embarrassment. An alternative is engaging in "mock" intimacy in very public settings. People will witness that a young woman is sexually or physically appealing to a man. The girl can flirt and screen out unacceptable partners without having behaved as if she were remotely interested in anyone for a more long-term involvement. The questions of who to trust and when to allow emotional intimacy are in part control issues. Young women who feel they have little control overall are most likely going to attempt to exercise a great amount of control in their private lives and to protect themselves from another layer of disappointment.

The Perfect Boyfriend

Though many boys make ideal "scoping" material and are considered potential casual sexual partners, only a subset are viewed as acceptable boyfriends. The expectations placed on potential boyfriends reflect a romantic ideal akin to the one previously noted by Elijah Anderson and others, but often the reality is different. Teenagers compromise on some of the nonnegotiable characteristics they seek in their ideal men in order to maintain any semblance of a committed relationship.

Regardless of family background, these teenagers have precise views of good and bad boyfriend material. This is one situation where the lines were clearly drawn and consistent. Good men are honest, emotional—yet not too emotive—generous, complimentary, observant, trustworthy, faithful, protective, and future oriented. Bad boyfriend material included men with too many relationships with "wrong" women. They are abusive, unfaithful, and unable to express intimate feelings; spent too much time with male friends; abused drugs/alcohol; and so on. However, in reality teenage girls constantly waffled on many of these declarations. If a boyfriend were at least five years her senior, a young woman might willingly ignore behavior she deemed totally unacceptable. Older men were a premium because they presumably earned more than teenage males, had more sexual and relationship experience, and were therefore more secure and willing to commit. Ultimately, what older boyfriends gave girls was an affirmation of their womanliness and femininity.

The question of fidelity often became transformed and was defined more fluidly by young women who discovered well into their relationships that their partners had strayed. Fidelity would be redefined as an established emotional connection, not physical and sexual exclusivity. This is particularly the case among teenagers who date well-known men, attractive men, and/or older men. The prestige and status inherent in *having been chosen* by such men is more important than demanding fidelity. These girls trade off one of the greatest romantic ideals for social recognition and respect. Men could "creep" or "mess around" as long as these encounters meant nothing on an emotional level. Although girlfriends do not want to be constantly reminded of their boyfriends' infidelity, they often resign themselves to the eventuality that it will occur. In part this behavior could be tolerated since the mythology surrounding male behavior included a resistance to sexual exclusivity.[21] Defining fidelity or faithfulness in this way means that some girls are exposing themselves to emotional stress and possibly health problems if the partner has many other unregulated sexual contacts.

Even the more cynical girls maintain the hope that the romantic ideal exists in the real world. They express distrust of men and disinterest in emotional ties yet often responded positively when female friends appeared to find a true romantic partner. They hold on to the belief that the perfect man may not be immediately available but may live outside the neighborhood, in a different kind of setting. Some plan to leave their communities in search of better lives; part of this search includes finding a strong relationship with a man.

Building a Relationship

In part what distinguishes a romantic relationship from a mere friendship is that others publicly recognize the new partnership. Finding an interesting partner is merely one stage in this relationship process. Getting the man to publicly acknowledge the relationship is essential. Young women realize that there are some peers who may express interest in them for purely sexual purposes. In these situations men may approach them in private or just in the presence of close friends. Once in a more open setting, the intimacy they experienced disappears.

> It is frustrating that some guys just don't really care what they do. They will promise you anything because they know that is what you want to hear. Then in the next breath they're acting like they don't even know you. I mean, I was talking to this one, and we're in his car, and at a light he sees some friends. And they come over and he says that he's giving me a ride home. That I'm just someone he ran into. Now here I am thinking that we're getting together. It isn't fair, that's all.

In this situation, the question of public boundaries is an issue. Public declarations of intention are meant to communicate commitment and also to warn others that the individual is unavailable.

In keeping with traditional roles, young women often did not confront their potential partner about the status of their relationship until some event occurred. The ritual of phone conversations, pagers, after school (as well as during) meetings, and time spent in a larger group set the stage for the development of the relationship. Young women expect that their boyfriends will pay attention to them and that this attention may require more time than their boyfriend wishes to spend. Tina's boyfriend is in his early twenties. He spent a few days on a trip with friends and promised to keep in touch while he was gone. When two days had passed without contact, she paged him. He did not respond to her page. A friend eventually told her that he was back in town, and she called his apartment. According to her, "he just needed some time on his own. He said he would have called me the next day. But he shoulda called when he got back. All he could say was that he doesn't have to report in. But he shoulda called me." In spite of her disappointment, Tina did not tell her boyfriend why she felt frustrated.

As Joyce Ladner (1995) discovered in her own field research, the girls who are most vocal about their boundary-setting expectations were older teenagers who have a more cautious view of men and relationships.[22] In some cases these girls had witnessed male-female confrontations while growing up. They had come to expect that men would not provide for them without being told what they must do. In other situations the girls had had experiences of their own that prompted them to "lay it all out for [the man]," as one teenager exclaimed. A third group of girls were the ones who did believe that men could maintain relationships. Though not cynical about men, they were more realistic about the prospect of romance. For them, love or commitment would not happen easily or quickly; these kinds of relationships would have to develop over time. They required "work, patience, and sometimes a smack upside the man's head." So the perceptions young women have of men, and how they intend to communicate with them, are as varied as the views held by adult women.

Making the transition from "talking" to exclusivity is at times complicated. Rarely did a young woman report that she and her partner discussed their relationship and their expectations of each other before making this transition. The intimacy found in close relationships developed as a result of spending greater amounts of time together. At that point, it was usually the young man who dictated the new parameters of the relationship. Sheree's experience was typical: "One day this girl said something about my boyfriend and I thought, 'Oh yeah—I guess that's what he is.' It's not like I didn't know; it just happened, kind of. At some point he said, 'You're my girl—all right?' and that was it." Although the establishment of the boyfriend–girlfriend relationship may be hazy, what transpires afterward is generally clear.

At some point the majority of teenagers in relationships deal with the issue of sex. Although not necessarily the primary purpose of a relationship, many girls anticipate that they will engage in sexual activity with their boyfriends. In fact, "[t]hose teenagers who have steady or regular partners are more likely to have premarital sex than are casual daters."[23] A steady partner connotes a kind of relationship in which kissing and holding hands are the means to an end, not ends in themselves. For some, sex is a way to express their love for their men. Others believe sex is a way to establish that the couple is involved in a relationship as opposed to just dating.

What is interesting, as I will discuss in the next chapter, is that there are many contradictions about the purpose and importance of sex with men. Some teenagers prefer to isolate sexual activity to relationships because of their need for affirmation, security, and validation. Others seek sex outside relationships for the same reason. So many young women prefer to have sexual intercourse outside a relationship because it will not lead to emotional intimacy. Without emotional intimacy they avoid possible rejection. As long as they are not rejected by men, their sexual identity is kept intact. For these young women, the promise of sexual involvement is not enough of a motivation for them to actively seek out a boyfriend. What the boyfriend *has* to offer them is emotional security and stability. In some instances girls with extensive sexual histories would only enter a relationship if their partner agreed to postpone sex. "This way," explained one nineteen-year-old mother, "if he's only in it for the wham bam, he won't wait around for very long. You get rid of the shallow, trifling ones right quick."

Commitment and Trust: What's Love Got to Do with It?

"I intend to marry the first man I fall in love with because that's the relationship that'll last," proclaimed one eighteen-year-old. "These young girls don't know the first thing about love." So, then, what do young women know about love, and is it a prerequisite for an intimate relationship? Romantic love is idealized on film, in novels, on television, and in popular magazines. Contrary to what some parents and other guardians may believe, young women have an understanding of love and commitment that is the union of some very sophisticated assessments and some youthful ones. They imagine a very idealistic interpretation of what the experience of love should be like. But this view is only in the realm of fantasy for them—it is what love should be like in theory. The reality of love and intimacy is not what they hoped to experience.

Older teenagers are on the whole more pragmatic in their view of what a relationship entails—especially those with children, who have seen both the best and the worst of what their boyfriends have to offer. Pamela is presently engaged to marry her boyfriend of over a year. When she met him at seventeen she already had a child. She had experienced an overwhelming amount of rejection from young men who were no more prepared for ready-made fatherhood than she had been prepared for pregnancy. Though in retrospect she understands and forgives them for their reactions, she recounts her anger at having been "booted" by "one man too many." Her initial response at the time was to

avoid any contact with these men. They gave me pain and heartache, and that was tiresome. I needed a real man, not someone who was all talk. I gave up on the chance at love. . . . Yeah, I know that sounds stupid, being that I was so young, but that's exactly how I felt. I figured I'd just take care of my baby as best I could and leave the rest in God's hands.

When she finally met George, Pamela wanted nothing to do with him. She believed that anyone expressing interest had an agenda. She had not given up the romantic ideal of love. She merely gave up on the possibility that she would experience it. The implications of her perspective were twofold. Pamela had a clear view of what an appropriate partner would have to offer; thus she was unwilling to acquiesce to what *could have been* a superficial gesture just to experience some form of love. Her relationship had to be interactive and symbiotic. Each person had to truly love the other.

Pamela, along with other teenage mothers, was world-weary when it came to love. Some, like her, decided to hold out for "the real deal." Others, however, gave up on their romantic ideal. These were the young women at risk of short-term sexual encounters. If there is no such thing as real adult love, then you must find love from either your children or from friendships. But because neither situation even approximates the feelings one experiences with romantic love, the logical conclusion is to maintain the only available element of intimate relationships—sex. A dose of cynicism is certainly apparent in this conclusion. Men are untrustworthy, yet they also offer no-holds-barred, noncommittal intimacy. Furthermore, they can provide you with children. Although young mothers who maintain this view like to claim that they do not need men, to some extent this opinion is simply inaccurate. They may not *need* men, but they want them. They may not marry, but they will bear a man's child. The child then represents both the love unavailable from their partner and the unconditional love of a baby.

Younger teenagers, especially those without children, are likely to equate their romantic ideal with reality. Romantic idealism is not normally associated with black teenagers, particularly poor ones. Some cloak their dreams in an attempt to appear streetwise and sophisticated. Reputation is of utmost importance, so the image of a love-sick girl is not one young women wish to represent. To outsiders they want to appear unconcerned with relationship building. Because they seem unconcerned about the implications associated with sexual activity, these girls are depicted in problematic ways. In this culture it is assumed that sexually active girls who are not in monogamous relationships must be cunning creatures who are comfortable using feminine wiles to get ahead. They are envisioned as carefree or callous about what they do with their bodies. They behave out of instinct and explain that "it just happened." Although impulse is definitely part of teenage sexuality, it is also very much a part of many adults' lives. For some reason, sexually active teenage girls bear the brunt of our collective social outrage and anger. In contrast, young women who date for a while before having sex, or who date and remain abstinent, are perceived as the only ones being sexually responsible—we assume that they are waiting to fall in love before becoming sexually intimate.

What many conversations illustrated was that these perceptions are very superficial and often wrong. Sexually active, nonmonogamous young women are often the ones who believe the most strongly in the romantic ideal. They look for love in every potential partner they meet and believe that each one is "the one." Sex becomes an instrument of their search for love. Time and again some of the most self-protective, seemingly ambivalent young women would reveal a vulnerable persona beneath the surface. They may use the language of independence and self-determination, but what they really wished for was a full-blown romance. Consider these observations: "I know we're in love because we are having a good time doing what we've got to do"; "He makes me feel so safe, it has to be love!" "I wanted him to know just what he means to me"; "I didn't want to lose him because he didn't feel what I thought he could feel." All four believed they were in love because they were having sex, and they presumed that real sex only occurs in romantic relationships.

Such a circular argument represents the traditional view of romance maintained by teenagers. It differs from the dysfunction we automatically associate with teenagers who have many partners. The irony here is that young women who envision themselves as being immune to romance and self-protective in actuality are risking rejection quite often and, more important, are jeopardizing their health. They express little trust of men yet expend a great amount of energy in search of a romantic "fix." They could appear to be fighting to retain control over their sexuality when in fact they really wish to relinquish control. Keep in mind that these young women hold fast to traditional views of gender roles and by extension traditional expressions of romance in relationships. By reifying what men are to do as well as how romance should feel, it becomes highly unlikely that the reality can ever be satisfactory. Men will never quite measure up and thus will bear the brunt of a woman's frustration and disappointment. For this reason some of the most cynical-sounding teenagers may in fact be romantic idealists.

In comparison, young women who abstain or limit their activity to one particular partner can be utilitarian and pragmatic in their view of sex. Such activity has to serve a purpose in their lives. Sex is not a means to an end but an end in itself. Sex is not what guarantees a love relationship. Instead, it symbolizes the culmination of an intimacy developed over time (whether over the course of a few weeks, months, or in some cases years). Romance is also a goal for these young women, but it appears to be less idealized in reality. "Boyfriends may or may not fall in love with you. . . . You can't force it to happen," one young woman told me. According to another one, "it's never good when you let a guy in too soon. If you do this and he isn't what you thought, then you gave away your virginity *and* you have to keep on without him." The quality of a relationship determines its potential for sexual intimacy. For middle-income girls or those with "middle-class aspirations," options are not reduced to "either I have sex, or there is no relationship."

Romance in the Realm of AIDS

Numerous researchers have recognized that women who value and act on traditional gender expectations and who have little power in a relationship are often at great risk for HIV infection because they are more willing to engage in behavior against their better judgment. Women who fear losing a boyfriend and who define themselves in terms of their partners are also likely to risk their health. Those who avoid developing relationships with a partner are at risk as well because they will either have many brief sexual encounters or don't trust their partner enough to take the time to learn about his sexual history. Romantic idealists may be at greater risk of infection than romantic pragmatists. Though there obviously is not causal connection between social class and relationship expectation, there may be a less formal link. For poor girls, the search for self control and autonomy becomes lost in the search for that one partner who will prove their mistrust of men wrong. The need to assert womanhood in the absence of alternate institutional means becomes associated with a recognition of femininity and sexuality.

Ultimately, personal and social elements will lead a young woman to define what kinds of relationships she is supposed to have, and she will behave accordingly. These definitions are rarely made self-consciously. Instead, they emerge as a result of a long process. Family, friends, and neighbors contribute to the parameters one creates regarding intimacy. A young woman will try on various personae until she finds one that suits her vision of who and what she should become. She will seek out partners who reflect her vision. As her life options change, so will her vision. What happens, then, to the young woman who see little opportunity for change in her future—what does she hold on to? She has her identity as a woman, which must be protected at all costs, even if this causes her to take risks.

5

Sexuality and Womanhood

The sexual revolution of the 1960s has been credited with permanently altering the sexual behavior of adults and youth in this country. Presumably, before this transformation in sexual mores, teenagers waited until marriage to become sexually active. Living with one's partner was inconceivable. Birth control was not readily available, and abortions were illegal. Sexually transmitted diseases were for the most part treatable or controllable. The extent to which contemporary attitudes regarding nonmarital sexual activity is a result of that era remains debatable. What is certain is that over the past three decades the number of teenagers with STDs and the number of unmarried teenagers who are parents have increased. Perhaps the reduction in pressure to marry young and the greater openness regarding sexuality may be at least partly responsible for these changes. Regardless of who or what has been the catalyst, the fact remains that every year teenagers are increasingly at risk for contracting HIV.

As health care professionals, counselors, and social scientists recognize, those who appear most likely to have sex while very young, become pregnant, and contract an STD are black youth.[1] At one time this reality led to some very punitive social policies aimed at regulating and controlling black sexual activity.[2] Some have claimed that black sexuality is fundamentally different from the sexuality of white, Asian, and Latino adults. In such arguments race supposedly explains differences in sexual activity and experience. This sort of "racial encoding" is reflected in research promoting images of the "natural sexual tendencies" of blacks.[3] Higher rates of sexual activity among young black teenagers are seen as evidence of this natural or genetic capacity for sex.

Obviously this position is inaccurate. First, it requires too broad sweeping a perception of black teenagers. Some, not all, are sexually active. Some engage in high-risk sex, but then so do teenagers from other racial-ethnic backgrounds. Second, by taking this generalized an approach, the connection between social class and sexual behavior is ignored. Poor white teenagers, particularly those in rural, isolated communities, are also likely to have sex while very young and to become pregnant. Middle-class teenagers, or those with the same view of the world as middle class youth, have more motives for delaying sex and avoiding pregnancy. So the question of the effects of race on sexual activity and HIV exposure also has to be approached from a social class perspective since there are both race and class differences in rates of sexual activity.

Although utilizing a more comprehensive race and class analysis is informative, it still leaves unanswered why teenagers even begin to have sex. Statistics show who is sexually active and presumably how often, but they cannot shed light on what these experiences are like, how sex might alter a young woman's perception of men in her life, or why young women abstain from sexual activity altogether. The observations and perceptions of the teenagers themselves occasionally provide views that are different from the ones implicit in the statistics. Race, economics, friendship, loneliness, self-acceptance, and so many other elements can influence the timing of a young woman's first, and often only, teenage sexual experience.

Sexuality in Adolescence

Sexual behavior involves more than a set of actions. It is infused with attitudes and beliefs, and previous experiences affect how one behaves sexually. Sexual behavior reflects the way an individual develops sexual attitudes, gender identity, and gender roles; it involves the acquisition of sexual skills, knowledge, and societal values.[4] Decisions regarding sexual activity are affected by a young woman's perception of power and control and by the meaning she attributes to womanhood.[5] Power, control, and progression toward adulthood are especially relevant concerns for teenagers who are negotiating new territory between childhood and adulthood.[6] Given all of this, adolescent sexuality is clearly somehow different from adult sexuality. But how? What makes teenage sexuality different from, and possibly more risk laden than, adult sexuality?

Raising this question places us in tricky territory. Agreeing that adolescent sexuality involves behavior that is unique does not mean that adolescent sexuality is fundamentally distinctive. Participation in high-risk sexual activity, from irregular or inconsistent condom use to multiple partners, is not the sole venue of teenagers. Adults engage in these actions as well. What is unique to adolescence is the way we perceive these behaviors. These perceptions reflect the universal belief that adolescence is a unique stage of development. Adolescence is a socially recognized category. Sex in adolescence is understood to be a manifestation of teenagers' need to experiment with social roles. What distinguishes adolescent sexuality is not what teenagers do but what motivates their behavior.

Adolescence is a modern concept that emerged during the Industrial Revolution.[7] As the purpose of the family changed, so did the roles of family members. Older members of the industrial and postindustrial family are responsible for both the financial and emotional well-being of the younger members. "Families are no longer primarily units of production and procreation; they have become instead centers of emotional and social support. Procreation is separated from sexual behavior and is an act of choice rather than necessity."[8] Adolescence, by the 1950s, was commonly considered a "sort of last bastion of youthfulness in our society . . . a period of general irresponsibility and confusion, a period in which people are quite immature and without substantial direction in their lives."[9] Adults view them as ill prepared to behave as adults, particularly in terms of interpersonal and emotional relationships with others.[10] These youth are biologically mature (i.e., they are able to reproduce) but not emotionally prepared to face the potential consequences of their behavior.[11] By the end of this period of transition, however, parents expect youth to begin manifesting the characteristics associated with adulthood: responsibility, maturity, and commitment to family and economic security. Upon entering adulthood, adolescents are permitted all the ensuing "trappings." This includes sexual activity.

Clearly, this is an idealized view; one not realized by many teenagers who *will* venture into some form of sexual activity. Some researchers have called this view of adolescence into question. For example, Anita Washington (1982) proposes that as a life stage adolescence is greatly affected by structural factors.[12] Members of poor communities perceive and treat teenagers as if they were adults much earlier than is traditionally expected. Having to assume financial responsibility, and being made privy to decisions normally relegated to adults are but two of the factors that result in the different treatment of poor youth. She further claims that if teenagers are treated as adults, they will face fewer sanctions for early sexual activity. This does not mean that in poor communities the youth are encouraged to quicken their march to adulthood but that rapidly maturing teenagers are not automatically labeled "problem youth" or "high risk."

Both Anita Washington's and Carol Levine's work provide useful insights that account for some of the demographic differences in sexual behavior among teenagers. They challenge the notion that teenagers undergo a unified, static process of development. Not all adolescents develop at the same speed physically—this we already know. What these authors illustrate is that these developmental differences may have sociological explanations. Both authors note that adolescence is as much a sociohistorical phenomenon as a psychological and physiological reality. In this century we have come to accept the notion that physical change occurs within discrete periods of time and that behavior changes as well. What life stage theorists contribute to this view is that the timing of and the importance placed on these changes varies. Broader social forces influence the timing of an individual's sexual activity and the course that it will take.

Sex, Social Class, and Race

There is some debate about the relative importance of teenagers' social class, peer norms, and sex-related knowledge on their sexual attitudes and sexual activity. In some studies, a teenager's decision to have sex is dependent on neither her peers' sexual attitudes nor her own views of what it means to be feminine.[13] However, other researchers argue the opposite.[14] For them, the average teenager deciding whether to have sex is certainly swayed by her perception of what peers do and the value they place on sexuality—both affect the development of a teenager's sexual identity and whether this developmental process results in sexual exploration. There is further disagreement about the effects of one's economic background on attitudes concerning premarital and early sexual activity. More specifically, the debate focuses on whether "[t]hese [economic and social] systems [that] generate social expectations, sanctions, and norms that influence and regulate fertility behavior . . . are subscribed to by both teens and their elders."[15]

Have these studies provided any common conclusions? With the exception of a minority of findings,[16] most indicate that early sexual behavior frequently occurs among teenage girls who consistently experience social inequality and isolation; these in turn affect girls' self-esteem and future-oriented life views.[17] Economic uncertainty, poor career opportunity, single-parent homes, and less concern for future options may lead to the initiation of sexual activity.[18]

Especially for poor teenagers, feeling isolated and unable to control the future results in declining interest in planning out or articulating preferred life goals and future plans. If "the system" has shown itself to be unreliable and if economic and personal success are considered to be correlated with particular class or ethnic groups, then teenagers who believe they are excluded from these avenues will also believe that they have little control over their lives. How economic conditions affect sexual behavior also has bearing on the ways in which teenagers are socialized to behave. Material reality shapes the social sphere in which a young woman learns about, and defines, her social roles and expectations. The power of gender, race, and class-based norms is that they can serve as self-fulfilling prophecies. A low-income black teenage girl and a middle-class black teenage girl have in common their race and gender. Each will at some point face barriers and challenges because of social position and the range of expectations associated with it. At the same time, though, the middle-class girl has opportunities and supports that just are not available to the poor teenager. What is important is that the experiences of more privileged girls instill in them the expectation that opportunities will always be available to them. Although a poor young woman wants to attain the same heights, she is more likely to assume that they will fall outside of her grasp. Thus, gender, class, and race all moderate behavior within the dominant society.[19]

Differences in sexual activity between whites and blacks are in large part explained by differences in the distribution of material resources and social support.[20] High incidences of sexual activity among blacks is partially a result of low socioeconomic status and high rates of urbanization.[21] Racial differences in sexual behavior are least apparent at higher levels of socioeconomic status (SES). A racially diverse group of teenagers from the same economic background will report very similar rates of sexual activity and pregnancy. In contrast, if one were to study the sexual activity of a racially homogeneous group of teenagers who come from varied economic backgrounds, she would discover variations in what they have experienced.

Joy Dryfoos (1990) has also confirmed that we need to consider the lasting effects of racial and economic inequality in order to understand why some black youth become sexually active.[22] Race and economic class are connected. The legacy of racism in this country has left a disproportionate number of black Americans poor. Children born into low-income households usually grow up poor. Parents teach them to anticipate racial and economic bias. At the same time, children are exposed to an array of messages coming from sources outside the home and community. Despite these parents' best efforts, some children conclude that they lack social value and thus lower what they expect in their futures. Teenagers in segregated, poor communities with declining employment opportunities maintain low expectations of school and work. Poor youth rarely see the fruits of academic labor within their community. They *do* witness and experience inequitable treatment within different social institutions, encounter more direct violence, and observe unpopular public images of people living in poverty. From this they conclude that few "outsiders" are willing to invest in their future. Among the societal factors still associated with delayed adolescent sexual activity are high educational achievement, social integration, supportive social conditions, and readily available employment.[23]

I found that these societal factors also influenced the actions of young women in New Haven. Understanding how opportunity affects sexuality requires considering how young women perceive their present lives. One such eighteen-year-old, Rhonda, lives in one of the poorest communities in New Haven with her parents and grandmother. Her first sexual experience of any kind, aside from kissing, was intercourse.

> When I was fourteen, I slept with my boyfriend. We had been going out for a few weeks and we were ready. . . . Oh, yeah, he was my first. My first boyfriend and my first sex. We had kissed before, and that was nice.

Laurine, who lives in the same area as Rhonda, also started with intercourse: "If I knew what I know now. Why get into it because we're in a hurry? So much else to have done . . . you know?" In contrast, seventeen-year-old Andie, from a middle-class family, dated her boyfriend for a few months before having sexual intercourse. In the period before they were first intimate,

> we couldn't keep ourselves in check. Messing around built things up. But we just wanted to chill for a while. It's a good thing since we broke up a while after. But we really took the time. That was good.

Low-income and poor teenagers of all races are the most likely to start their sexual lives early in a relationship. The fact that there is a general difference among young women from various economic backgrounds regarding sexual activity is only part of the story. What is also interesting is the way all young women categorize, define, and differentiate sexual activity. Sometimes the pursuit of sex is actually the pursuit of closeness. For other young women, sex guarantees the presence of men in their lives. Certain sexual activity is unacceptable to some, while "normal" to others. There is as much variety of opinions among teenagers as there is among adults. At the same time, however, some general trends in the extent of sexual activity do exist.

Which Teenagers Are Having Sex?

More men and women under the age of eighteen are having sex than during virtually any other decade in history. Rates of sexual activity have been rising progressively over the past two decades. This increase is partly due to more liberal public attitudes concerning premarital sex, the rapid physical and sexual maturation of teenagers, and the availability of affordable contraception. Approximately 74 percent of teenagers will have intercourse by the time they are nineteen.[24] If the definition of sexual activity is expanded to include any form of physical contact between partners—anything from fondling to intercourse—then about 85 percent of teenagers will experience some form of sexual activity before turning nineteen.[25] The average teenage female first has sexual intercourse at sixteen. Starting to engage in intercourse at this age does not mean that she will continue to have sex throughout adolescence. In actuality, most teenage girls have intercourse very infrequently. Although this observation means that the risk of HIV infection is somewhat lessened, the specter of risk still remains. It only takes one encounter to contract HIV or become pregnant.

Young women who report frequent sexual activity first experience sex at a younger age: between fourteen and fifteen years of age.[26] These young women appear to value their independence and freedom even more than other teenagers. They are more tolerant of nontraditional sexual beliefs and behavior. Most do not believe that an education or economic stability is available to them because these fall outside the range of things they can control. In contrast, young women who delay sexual activity until their late teens have higher educational and career aspirations, believe that they have control over their lives, and express comfort with discussing sexual issues with their mothers and partners.[27]

The typical perception of young black women's sexual activity is that they engage in it early and often. This is only true for some young black girls. In actuality, the rate of sexual activity among white teenagers has increased at least twice as rapidly as the rate among black teens.[28] During the past two decades, the gap between black and white teenagers' rates of sexual activity has narrowed. Fifty-two percent of white young women have had intercourse compared with 60 percent of black and about 50 percent of Latina teenagers. White teenage girls are having sexual contact with teenage boys at increasingly younger ages. What is interesting to note is that the kinds of sexual behavior young black women experience differ from those of their white and Latina counterparts. As we shall see, this variation will help us to understand the different rates of STD infection among these three groups of young women.

Young white women start sexual experimentation at about the same time as black teenage women, but what they actually do is very different.[29] Before initiating intercourse, Caucasian girls experience what is called "nonprocreative" sexual activity much more frequently than blacks. They experiment with "petting," oral sex, and anal sex. Sexual activity occurs in stages: first kissing, then petting, heavy petting, and eventually intercourse. White teenagers generally initiate intercourse later in adolescence, so the window of opportunity during which they face HIV infection and teenage pregnancy is narrow. However, once they do experience intercourse, young white women have more sexual partners than black teenagers. These sexual relationships are referred to as "serially monogamous" relationships, which means that young white women have a succession of monogamous contacts. Multiple partnering places these young women at a high risk of HIV infection.

Young black women experience foreplay much less often than white teenagers.[30] They tend to initiate intercourse after only a brief period of nonprocreative activity (petting). In fact, they report having sexual intercourse two to three years before young white women. As a result, black teenagers face the risk of both contracting HIV and becoming pregnant for a longer stretch of adolescence. Even after becoming sexually active, few report experiencing other forms of sexual behavior. This raises interesting issues. Though many teenagers of all racial and economic backgrounds will be sexually active at some point, not all of them will engage in the same kinds of behaviors. On average, black teenage girls start having sex young but ultimately have fewer sexual partners than white females. Obviously sex does not mean the same thing to all young women.

According to case workers and educators I interviewed, the majority of black girls they encountered were sexually active and had started having sex very young. Though they suspect that the majority of young women have had sex at least once, counselors also suspected that some teenagers may overreport how frequently they have sex because the teenagers are aware of the popular perception of black sexual activity. The majority of young women I met said that they had been sexually active and that they had become so at a young age. Over half of the women who have had sex first did so before the age of sixteen. Many of them mentioned having intercourse with an older male, over twenty-one, and stated that they first learned about sex from friends or their partners. The young woman who initiates sexual activity, particularly before the age of fifteen, is one who feels some social isolation, whose life options (in her view) are limited. For her, sex—from the choice of partner to the timing of sexual encounters—is one kind of behavior that could not be denied her by either individuals or institutions such as school and church. Love, while a romantic ideal, is not a prerequisite or a by-product of sexual relationships. While they are for the most part ambivalent about being sexually active, they also articulate that intercourse is a means of retaining and wielding power in their personal relationships.

Teenagers who abstain from sexual intercourse are more comfortable with their sexuality; femininity and womanhood are not synonymous with sexual activity. It is easy for them to resist any sort of sexual peer pressure they may encounter. Ironically, they are as concerned about retaining control over their lives as sexually experienced young women, but their motivation is quite different. They believe that romantic relationships can be developed and are thus willing to "wait for the right one." Most may not express an interest in abstaining until marriage, but they do intend to take their time developing a relationship before engaging in sex. Sexual intercourse is not a necessity for the girls who delayed intercourse or were monogamous. Again, the effects of SES are apparent. Given that these girls perceive more opportunities in their future and believe that regardless of external barriers they can attain those goals, the potential importance of intercourse is tempered. In a sense it is decentered in their lives. It becomes one of many different activities they can consider. They can afford not to have sex because they have other life-affirming opportunities.

Throughout discussions, certain themes emerged. Intimacy was important to all of the young women but was sought through different means. For ones who delayed intercourse, relationships with families and partners were already emotionally intimate. These girls trusted the men in their lives and expected to build a close bond in their relationships. Intercourse was not a necessary source of emotional intimacy. Young women who engaged in sex at young ages also sought intimacy, but through intercourse. Even so, they did not expect to develop an intimate relationship with their partner because so few trusted men or their potential stability. Emotional commitment and long-term intimacy require trust, time, and patience. Sex was a way to experience intimacy without commitment or the risk of partner loss.

Sexual Expectations and Experiences

Teenagers under sixteen conceptualize sex as a spontaneous, romantic event that would occur with someone they love. Sharing sexual love with a partner is more important than considering their own readiness for the experience. Even sexually active younger teens maintain a romantic view of their sexuality. This disclosure was not forthcoming in early discussions, when the teens I met were more concerned with controlling their images and with appearing stronger and more independent to me. After some time, I began to notice a trend in the ways they talked about sex, as if the mystery surrounding the act itself were intact.

> **TM:** Being with him is so beautiful. Now we are close. We like to do it whenever we can, 'cause we like each other. Well, we sort of love each other. I know he loves me, and I love him too, so it is okay. I can't think of how things would be if we didn't do the thing.
> **RTW:** When did you know you were in love with him? How did you know?
> **TM:** When I wanted to . . . you know . . . be with him. That meant I had to love him, didn't it?
> **RTW:** I don't know. If you didn't have sex, would you still feel love for him?
> **TM:** Yeah, 'cause he's cool. But now I know for sure that we're in love because of the sex. He loves me even more too. At least that what he says all of the time. And since he's almost twenty, he knows what he talks about. That's how it is.

Sex represents commitment and love, not sexual pleasure, desire, or autonomy. Few of these younger teenagers describe sex as pleasurable or essential in their lives. In fact, most are sexually active because (1) their partner has expressed interest in it; (2) once they start, they are afraid of suddenly stopping and losing their partner; or (3) they are afraid that if they stop, they will never grow to like it.

Though sensitive to how others responded to their behavior, sexually active teenagers were less concerned than abstinent teens about others' assessments of their behavior. A few conflicting elements are at work. First, young women with an extensive sexual history became active to attain adult status. If they felt more mature or sophisticated because of their sexual activity, they were likely to express satisfaction with themselves. It would not be inconsistent, then, for surveys to indicate that sexually active girls score high on positive self-image while scoring low on measurements of their level of comfort with their sexuality.[31] This contradiction is reflected by many who report regret over the timing of their initial sexual activity while claiming to be satisfied with having become sexually experienced.

Among older teenagers, sexuality is as important as the act of sex. Although love and commitment are important, they are not necessary for either engaging in or enjoying sex. In conversations, they told me that pleasure, control over sex, responsibility for birth control, vocal assertion with partner(s), and sexual compatibility were very important issues for them. Most with this perspective were teenage mothers. All but one were also poor or working poor. Not depending on a man for social and emotional support reduced his potential role in their lives and increased their responsibility for their sexuality within a relationship.[32]

Being sexually active is not the same as being sexual. I believe that we often confuse the two, especially when discussing adolescent sexuality. Engaging in sexual activity neither causes nor is caused by a young woman's comfort with herself as a sexual being. Young women express discomfort with the physiological changes in their bodies. Although they may know what is happening and what it symbolizes, they are rarely happy with the changes. Some of the most sexually sophisticated young women would do anything to avoid discussing specific biological functions. They were either ambivalent or embarrassed by this proof of their sexuality. In this exchange, Angela attempted to explain how her reproductive and other physiological functions changed during puberty:

Angela: First you grow, then you can get pregnant, then you have a few kids. It's the usual story.

RTW: Does anything happen between growing and getting pregnant?

Sharon [another participant]: Yeah, Miss Smart Thing. What happens? [laughter in background]

Angela: Hormones go wild around . . . what's it called? Pub. . . .

Sharon: -erty. P-U-B-E-R-T-Y. Get it together.

Angela: So, I got that [gestures to her breasts] for about the past three years. They ain't big, but boys like them anyway. Now, the blood—you know, my period—started about the same time. I think it's nasty, but now I can have babies, so that's cool. I know I get that syndrome thing, 'cause at that time I can be a real bitch. Now I'm looking too good for words, and I like the way it makes men look at me. My girlfriend Larissa don't got any of it yet, and she's fifteen, like me! I try to tell her not to feel bad, but I don't know what I'd do if I was still looking like a child.

RTW: Why do you think she hasn't started her period yet?

Angela: Like I said, there's something goin' on way inside of her. She ain't working right. Her insides must be all scrambled up like an egg [laughs]. Not too funny, I guess, but of all my girlfriends, she's the one who wouldn't have it yet. She don't like boys. I mean, she isn't one of those kind; she just don't care about boys, so she isn't needing her period for anything.

Sharon: Oh, come on, Angela, you don't really believe she hasn't got her period because of that, do you? I didn't get mine till I was fifteen, and there sure isn't a thing wrong with me! Maybe she just isn't supposed to yet, you know.

Angela: I know how things work, okay! Your chemicals get all mixed up, and then you start to bleed once a month. Your body gets different and you can get pregnant. That's all you need to know. That's all I want to know.

Even though there is a range of difference in the depth and accuracy of their knowledge of reproductive functions, what many of the group had in common was an unwillingness to be specific about their biological and physical changes. For these young women, sexual knowledge did not necessarily translate into comfort with physical characteristics associated with sexuality and gender.

Those who are more likely to know about ovulation and hormonal changes are women whose parents started talking about sex when they were young. Young women whose families educated them at a young age came from middle- and lower-middle-class families. Additionally, the most vocal about their own bodies were, not too surprisingly, also the most comfortable with their appearance. Self-esteem and self-love are often associated with feeling comfortable with one's sexuality. This esteem, according to the literature in social psychology, is most often instilled by family and maintained through a supportive and loving social network.[33] Teenagers who had delayed sexual intercourse until after sixteen were more comfortable with their sexuality than young women who had experienced some sexual activity. What this raises is the relationship among self-esteem, delayed sexual behavior, and beliefs and perceptions concerning sex.

Few young sexually active women were comfortable with their sexuality. Girls frequently describe strong feelings of guilt. Although they believe being sexual is important, they dislike sex, and they appear uncomfortable with their sexuality. Why this conflict between feelings and behavior among younger, childless, sexually active teenagers? In talking about sex, they are generally more easily influenced by their peers and do not view themselves as able to resist the pressure to have sex. They have had minimal access to ongoing conversations with their parents or guardians about being sexual. The meaning they attach to sex is less defined by how they feel than by how their partner feels. Older teenagers' perceptions are naturally the result of having more experience to reference and of being more resistant to peer pressure.[34]

Virginity

What do teenagers really feel about sex, and how important is it to their personal relationships? In part, young women's opinions of virginity can shed light on these questions. Discussions of sex and self-esteem allude to teenagers' guilt feelings about sex but have not explicitly broached the subject of the "value" of virginity.[35] Teenagers do not view male virgins and female virgins in the same way.[36] I noticed that a double standard persisted among most of the teenagers about what male and female virginity "meant." As one young girl said, "I would never go with a virgin. If he hasn't had anyone yet, I'd wonder whether there was something funny about him." In contrast, though, she did not question female virgins' sexuality: "If a girl can last that long, more power to her. Guys are so persistent that she'd have to be pretty strong to stay one."

Virginity is a gift to be saved for marriage. Even teenagers who are virgins and intend to remain that way until marriage acknowledge that they are the exception rather than the rule. I asked one sixteen-year-old, a devout Catholic, whether she was uncomfortable identifying her sexual status to other girls and potential boyfriends:

> Not really, because I know deep down that what I'm doing is right. I'd bet that most of those girls who have lots of sex will be sorry later on. For me, making a decision about sex is too important to make on a whim. As far as boys, well, it really isn't any of their business what I plan to do. If they like me, they have to respect my opinion, or else they're out of here. Honestly, I think girls think it's kind of neat that I'm a virgin. I'm some kind of relic or something—like a dinosaur! Some boys want to date me to devirginize me and stuff, but I won't let them. I have to be married.

Another young woman, fifteen, feels similarly:

> Sometimes I almost think it'd be easier to just get it over with and do it. Then I think about all sorts of things, like, "what if he's a jerk?" and "it's going to hurt so much." Then I'm okay. I believe that you have to be really in love to begin with, you know, before you start. I'll probably be more comfortable with the thought of sex when I'm older, like eighteen or nineteen.

Among the young women who have never experienced anything sexual (including heavy petting), religion is not the most common reason they offered. Most stated that they chose not to have sex because they felt they were too young to manage the potential negative outcomes (including contracting an STD or becoming pregnant).

Virginity has many meanings to young women. For some, it is a trophy to be won or earned by a man. For others, it merely represents childhood and is an impediment to becoming mature. Being called a virgin or appearing "virginal" is an insult that is akin to being called immature or unworldly by one's peers. It is commonly viewed as a negative personality trait, as a quality that is intrinsic to one's identity, or as a burden.

These perceptions of virginity are at odds with the way sexually active teenagers viewed young women they believed were virgins. Even those teenagers who were critical of preserving one's virginity did not disapprove of the choice to abstain but rather the possible outcomes. According to Reed, a sixteen-year-old, "there's no point in keeping it [virginity]. I think that girls who won't have sex are just dumb. If they don't give it up, what do they think, that the guy will wait around? Get real—he'll find someone else." Teenagers who most often valued virginity were older ones who had reported extensive sexual activity (having had intercourse with at least five partners). Although they might not regret becoming active, some of this cohort regretted how, when, and with whom their first sexual encounters occurred.

There is tension between the image of the virgin and the value of virginity. Young virgins are respected for their choice to abstain but are considered less mature because of their inactivity. Sexual activity is closely tied to the image of a woman—to being a woman. Being able to attract a man with one's body is important, but the sexual intercourse is rarely enjoyed. Once she is sexually active, a teenager enters the realm of adulthood in the opinion of her peers. Virginity is associated with great internal strength and spirituality, but having these traits as an abstainer does not result in their being identified as womanly or adult since virginity is not respected.

Defining Sex

Some young women define sex solely in terms of intercourse. A few even claimed they did not realize there was anything outside of kissing and intercourse. As Deanna explained:

> When you're talking with your girlfriends about what you want to do, or what they do, or anything, you never say anything about those other things. I mean, why waste time with things that don't get to the point? He's there for one thing, and so am I, so why not get into it? . . . Especially at a party, when you meet your man, and there's not much time, or something.

Deanna identifies an important social setting where sex occurs—parties. In these settings, sociability plus alcohol lead to sexual encounters. Teenagers have intensive extended contact with each other, but the space and time for sexual activity are limited. With sex so immediately available, there are limited chances for using certain forms of birth control. Sponges, diaphragms, and even condoms become cumbersome—if sex is imminent, who is going to stop willingly in order to find a condom? Spontaneous sex brings with it the increased possibility of unprotected and thus risky sex.

Numerous teenagers described their first few sexual encounters as rushed and devoid of any emotional connection with the partners. In their view, the men were only interested in their own gratification. According to Barbara, "a man wants nothing that don't have to do with his dick. And his dick just wants one thing. So that's all he gets." Often poor girls had intercourse early in their relationships because they were afraid of losing their boyfriend/partner, because they were curious and believed the sex would eventually improve, or in some cases because sex was "a way to kill time when there's nothing on cable."

Sexual activity outside intercourse only should involve a trusted, close partner. Public health officials might identify some of these activities (such as manual stimulation) as low risk, but in actuality teenagers perceive them as emotionally high risk. Both active and abstinent young women believe that romantic or emotionally intense sex involves exploration and intimacy. However, for sexually active and socially isolated young women, sexual exploration is time-consuming and requires an interest in and commitment to developing a relationship with "strings" and expectations. Again we can see how defining intercourse as a quick path to intimacy without risk leads to this perception. This still leaves unanswered the need to define intercourse as more essential to quick intimacy than other sexual behaviors.

Young women who feel they have no other outlets through which to experience intimacy are the ones most likely to seek it through sex. In contrast, young women who avoid or abstain from sex are the least likely to need intercourse for intimacy. They are also more likely to believe that they can maintain some control over their lives. What this point implies is that women who fear losing control in their relationships seek spontaneous intimacy with men because anonymous or acquaintance sex requires little emotional investment and vulnerability.

For those socially alienated young women who feel disassociated from others and who are barred from traditional modes of adult behavior, intercourse becomes synonymous with sexuality, maturation, and power/control. Sexual activity is clearly linked with maturity and adulthood. Physical changes are proof of biological and chronological maturation. Being able to attract men and sexually satisfy them is evidence of sexual maturity. Having an older boyfriend is incontrovertible evidence that one is truly a woman. One of the lessons learned while growing up is that sexual activity is reserved for adults and those rare teenagers who are emotionally prepared for the ramifications of their behavior. Even though there is truth to this message, an unintended effect is that adolescents who want to grow up quickly may opt for intercourse.

Among younger sexually active girls, oral sex and other behavior were unacceptable because they represented too much closeness; "once you've seen his thing," explained one sixteen-year-old, "you don't want to be with him any more. I never knew how nasty it was. Now you say I should have that thing in my mouth? *That* is not my kind of thing."[37] Combined with the expectation that sexual intercourse leads to becoming an adult, it becomes apparent that for young women who do not expect to be adults (by living long enough or achieving the trappings of adult success), early intercourse can satisfy various needs.

If sex and intercourse are identical for a teenager and if she is starting to have intercourse early in her reproductive years, then a range of related risks begin to emerge. This is particularly true if part of her motivation is to keep or please an older boyfriend and not to satisfy her own needs. Many young women who had had sex very young reported that their first partners were older men. Young women with adult partners defined intercourse as a necessary intimacy-building experience because their partners set the parameters for their sexual relationships. These women recognized that their boyfriends wanted intercourse and that if they refused, these men would seek other young women. Furthermore, though not necessarily looking for a "loving" relationship (because of fear of emotional abandonment and vulnerability), these girls did want intimacy from sexual contact. Intercourse becomes defined as a low-risk intimacy. For teenagers who postponed intercourse, intimacy comes from the development of a relationship first and then possibly from a wider range of sexual behaviors. This time-consuming and emotionally risky process is not problematic for them since they are less likely to draw their self-image from either their partner or from sex. Time is not an enemy, and sexuality is not equated with femininity or womanhood.

Teenagers from emotionally supportive and financially stable households tend not to equate sex and intercourse. Other means of expressing their sexual identity before intercourse are available. Postponing the timing of intercourse until late adolescence and minimizing the risk of pregnancy and contracting STDs is a realistic option. Is it possible that the definition of sex as a range of behaviors (including, but not restricted to, intercourse) is somehow a gatekeeping or social control mechanism that encourages middle-class teenagers to postpone sexual intercourse? Perhaps if sexuality is commonly defined in broader parameters than intercourse, teenagers would be equipped with the perspective that late-adolescence sexual intercourse will be accepted by peers. Such a viewpoint allows them to be sexual without risking their educational and professional development. Though studies emphasize that white teenagers are generally more likely to experiment with oral sex and other activity before intercourse, I met middle-income black teens who are also likely to do so. In fact, middle-class black teenagers reported avoiding any activity that might lead to intercourse, especially oral sex.

Distinguishing between intercourse and other kinds of intimate activity was not the result of religious training or any overall commitment to remaining virgins until marriage. Recognizing that other sexual options are possible is important to young women who want to find activities that express intimacy and commitment to their partner while still avoiding the risk of pregnancy (and, to a lesser extent, contracting an STD). Julia, who has been with her boyfriend for approximately a year and a half, reflects the sentiments of others in her social class when she said:

> I like hanging out with Robert. There's always something to do with him. . . . We mainly kiss and stuff. I don't get into anything else. I like [professional basketball player] David Robinson's attitude. If you know you care about someone and want to be with them, why not focus on that rather than sex? If you avoid any situation where clothes are coming off, you're better off. Even though I care about Robert, I don't think I'm ready for the whole thing yet. Anyway, who knows if we can handle the responsibility of sex, or even worse, a baby?

For girls such as Julia, sex was not intimacy, and intercourse did not signify maturity or adulthood. On the contrary, these middle-class girls consistently believed that they needed to be mature *before* they would be ready to engage in intercourse. For example, young women voiced concerns over their ability to withstand the emotional pressures that come with initiating intercourse, in addition to the possible risks of pregnancy and contracting an STD. As a result of these two realizations, intercourse had to be avoided in order for them to develop mature, close, and trusting relationships with their partners. Only this kind of relationship could withstand intercourse.

Alternate activities did not carry the physical and emotional risks inherent in intercourse. These activities were often not sexual in nature:

> Too much is going on in the world to make me think of sex. There's more to life than having an orgasm, you know. . . . I enjoy spending time with

a guy. If you rush into sex, what do you think others will think of you? Especially if you don't know him well. I'm in no hurry.

I go to movies a lot. I mean, we do. I hang with friends, go to parties. Stuff in that mind-set, you see? My man is as fine as they come, so I'm sure folks think we have sex. I would like to at some point, but we have lots of time. Why rush? I figure if he wants me for me, he'll wait for the sex.

For both young women, stable relationships with men are not be dependent on intercourse—they have foreseen the possibility of becoming close to young men without engaging in sex.

Some of the teenagers with whom I spoke directly addressed the distinction between sexual intercourse and other sexual activity. Consider Gerry, for example, who described when she will plan on having sex in her relationship:

Sex could happen, but not right away. Not that we don't mess around though, because we do. A lot. I believe we could get more intimate, but there is no pressure at the time being. We are getting more comfortable with each other now. I know what he likes, and he makes me happy.

She has defined categories of acceptable sexual behavior that are similar to the popular baseball analogy in which bases correspond to various levels of sexual involvement. Gerry strongly believes that "making out" has to occur for some time before she would consider "going further, as far as actual sex."

Other factors influenced the way middle-class teenagers perceived sexual intercourse. This young woman sees intercourse as a possibility but is concerned with how her image would be affected:

I really want to sleep with him [new boyfriend], but I could see things getting carried away. I thought about preparing, with a nice dinner and all of that, but then I think about whether he'd respond in the way I want. If I initiate, does that make me too pushy or something? I wonder. . . .

Differences between black and white teenagers' sexual behavior can be understood as the result of the ways social class affects the development personal relationships, the need for intimacy, and the expectations teenagers set for their relationships with men. Class, through the imposition of opportunity structures and other rigid social barriers, mediates the way poor black teenagers are devising strategies for emotional survival and independence while still seeking intimacy and closeness.

Sex and Pregnancy: Fast Tracks to Adulthood?

Sustained, consistent economic development in urban areas and stable teen employment rates enable teenagers to make the transition to adulthood easily and to maintain positive life prospects. Without the combination of these family, personal, and community variables, teenagers are susceptible to engage in early and risky intercourse.[38] Negative perceptions of future life options, minimal sanctions for teen sex, and increased susceptibility to peer pressure are associated with poverty, which in turn is correlated with early sexual behavior.

How are these elements played out in the lives of poor teenagers? Within socially and materially impoverished communities throughout the United States, long-term relationships with men are elusive. By their early twenties many men are incarcerated, dead, or uninterested in permanent relationships.[39] Too many young women literally watch the men in their community die on a daily basis to believe in permanent relationships or long-term economic support from one man. Love and commitment become as fantastic as departure from their neighborhood. Economic security, career growth, and social mobility remain unreachable.[40] A more realistic and controllable situation is determining the contexts in which sex can be experienced. Even if other arenas in their lives cannot be controlled, they can still enjoy control over sex and how their sexuality affects men.

By making this argument, I do not intend to imply that these young black women are either manipulative or "highly" sexual—merely that they clearly distinguish sex from intimacy and trust. One explanation for the common perception that the act of sex is a commodity to be manipulated or withheld is that some young women do not and will not trust young men. This view is exemplified by teenage mothers who raise their children alone.[41] In addition to facing the scrutiny of social service agencies, they also have to face life without the child(ren)'s father. Few men in poorer communities have either the means or an emotional commitment to raising other people's offspring.

Sharon, a working-class nineteen-year-old with two children ages twenty months and four years old, expressed strong distrust of men. She had dated the father of her eldest child for over a year before she became pregnant. She remembered avoiding telling him until she was well into her second trimester, thinking that by being so far along, he would be more inclined to support her throughout the remainder of her pregnancy. Instead:

The motherfucker just looked at me and says, "So? What am I supposed to do with somebody's kid?" *Somebody's* kid? Who the hell do he think he is? Just fuck me, love me, and that's the end? So I tell him I'm fine on my own, don't need his bullshit anymore. I have DeSharon anyway, and I survive. . . . Then there's Tawn's dad. At least he stuck with me till after the labor. And some after that. But he couldn't take the stress of having a baby and needing to give me money. He screwed up, like a guy, but he tried for a while. So I figure, what's up with these men, you know? I got my babies, don't need their shit either. Can't even stay the night or nothing. It's just "thanks, and get out!"

In later conversations, Sharon shared with me more of her philosophy concerning relationships with men: "I like to party, but I don't look for any more. These guys can't give any more than that. Don't sweat this. Just have a little fun, no pain, no hurt."

Among young women who have their children's father in their lives, a modicum of distrust still exists. Their general sense is that relationships have the potential to be transient, or at least tenuous. Common phrases in our discussions included "I know I got my man, but . . ." and "You never know for sure about a man." Even among women who declare that their partner is completely reliable and monogamous, fear still persists of other women's potential influence. Often, the discussion turns to identifying the "skeeze" or "ho" who challenged their relationships. Interestingly, there is little concern over selecting men who believe in monogamy because the common assumption is that men cannot control their sexual drive and thus are intrinsically unreliable. The emphasis is on minimizing contact with women who have been identified as sexually liberal or promiscuous. Therefore, women who are considered threatening receive the bulk of other women's anger.

These same attitudes are expressed when discussing sexual assault and violence. The most common statistics indicate that as many as one out of every four women will be subjected to sexual assault in her lifetime.[42] What is as striking is the number of young women in this study who have been coerced into sexual activity. Particularly those who identify their relationships as committed report what they consider to be excessive pressure to have sex with their partner or his friends. Although aware of the implications of their partners' behavior, they justify these actions as being expected within the framework of a romantic partnership or as being "natural" behavior among men:

We were chillin' out for a while and then started to mess around. I knew that he wanted to do it, but I wasn't feeling good, and just wanted to take it easy. . . . He got pissed and was going to walk . . . so we end up doing it. He just couldn't wait, you know? Maybe I shoulda been stronger, but he got what he wanted anyway. Got hot pants. Was pushy and all; I shoulda been stronger. They always want it, all the time, so what else is new, right?

This seventeen-year-old young woman had been involved with her partner for two years and described numerous situations when he would physically force her to engage in some sexual activity with him. She appears aware that this behavior was unacceptable but either passed it off as "typical boy's stuff" or argued that rape or coercion could never occur in a long-term relationship.[43] The most common coercion experienced by these teenagers consisted of young men reminding them that there were few available and acceptable young men to date. Consequently, if one woman is unwilling to have sex, many others remain who will. This strategy is identified in communities where the young men are at greater risk of incarceration or early death.[44]

Is sex a signifier of maturity? Concern over control and opportunity, and feelings of alienation, can be resolved through sex. The short-term benefit is immediate closeness with someone. If men may not remain in one's life, the solution is to access them whenever and however one can. Naturally this view contradicts the perception that freedom in sexual activity means not depending on men. At the same time, though, it is the perfect expression of independence. Not creating ties with men is a choice, just as pursuing them for sex is a choice.

Older sexual partners are evidence of maturity, at least in the eyes of the teenager in the relationship. More important, older men also offer more security and knowledge than younger men. Deena believes that older men are more valuable because "they have more money to spend on you and your children. They have more to give and want to because they get some young thing in return." For Jasmine, older men "like acting like they're all that. As if I don't know shit myself. I can't stand that. Sometimes you get one who'll treat you real nice and do things a different guy wouldn't know how to do." Being treated differently, feeling pampered, and experiencing fundamental feelings of acceptance can all come from dating older men. Part of the benefit is a young woman knowing that she "won out over these other women."

Although none of the teenagers I met ever expressed this opinion, many saw sex as a way to appear grown up. Having an older man interested in them, being able to choose from a variety of interested men, or changing partners became symbolic of adulthood. Appearing in control, possessing material rewards from sexual relations— signified by a good boyfriend who "buys lots of good things, like clothes"—or getting pregnant and seeing one's body as a reflection of womanhood are all ways sexual activity, and thus sexuality, become identified as alternate routes to adult status.

Pregnancy and parenthood are traditionally adult experiences. For teenagers who wish to hasten their entry into adulthood, parenthood becomes one feasible means of doing so. Though experiencing some pressure from friends to behave as adults, these teenagers are also responding to the social definition of what adulthood and maturity mean—namely, parenthood. During subsequent conversations, Rhonda told me that she was pregnant with her first child. She explained that having her child would make her feel special, in a way she had not expected:

> **Rhonda**: Every time I feel him move, I know I've done the right thing. My man wanted me to get rid of him, but how can I? This baby needs a grown-up and I'm all he has.
>
> **RTW**: Why do you say you're all he has?
>
> **Rhonda**: Well . . . there are some people but I'm his mom. That's what it's all about. Being a mother.
>
> **RTW**: Do you think you were a responsible person before . . .
>
> **Rhonda**: You mean the baby?
>
> **RTW**: Yes.
>
> **Rhonda**: But this is different. He looks up to me. That's going to be fun. He needs a grown-up. His mother.

In considering what pregnancy, parenthood, and childbirth represent to teenagers, we need also to consider how these issues are valued in a wider social framework.

In spite of the current reality for most mothers, who work outside of the home and are still expected to assume the bulk of household responsibilities, mother as a symbol remains mystified.[45] Young men and women are subject to these conflicting images of mother and the tendency to subsume woman under the heading of maternal.[46] "There is something about being pregnant that is so beautiful," explained Gina. "Being a mother is great." When I asked her to explain why motherhood is so appealing, she said, "Look at me. I'm fat and happy. People respond to me more now than at any other time!" Getting attention and being valued for her pregnant state were extremely important for Gina. As a biologically determined category, female as childbearer easily becomes confused with the social construction of femininity and womanhood (i.e., a chronological stage that is distinct from girl and teenager).

> Reproduction is not simply a biological process. Women do not breed like cows. . . . [W]omen have in the past experienced and observed their reproduction, and passed on the knowledge they have gained to their

daughters. Women's experiences of the productivity of our whole bodies affect who we are, and how we relate to the world. This is not a biologistic argument, that is, one that reduces women's behavior to biology. It is a rejection of the false split between the "purely" biological and the social. It is an affirmation of women's sensuous reproduction and our bodily existence in the world.[47]

In her challenge to traditional notions of womanhood, Patricia Spallone (1989) examines the gray area among conceptions of sexual identity, gender, and reproduction. Though she is convincing in her observation, I doubt that many teenagers would successfully understand the links she notes between the biological and socially constructed definitions of woman and mother.

In addition to being a role assigned certain expected behaviors, motherhood is also a social status. Marlene is preparing for college in a year and has decided to wait a few years before having children.

> I definitely plan to have a family. I respect mothers. Now that I am older, I can see what hard work it is. I help my mom with my little brother, so I have a sense of what's involved. I think when I have had more real-life learning I could make a good mother.

Marlene is as respectful of motherhood as young women who became pregnant. What distinguished her, and others, from young mothers is that she does not need motherhood to improve her social status. She explained further: "I love children and like playing with them, but that's enough of a responsibility for now."

In being connected with adulthood, maturity, and womanhood, pregnancy and motherhood assume greater meaning. As a social status, motherhood is identified with a change in location within the general social hierarchy.[48] This is especially powerful for teenagers who see no other ways to gain respect from others. In one eighteen-year-old's view:

> Since having my kids, people know not to mess with me. I have too much going on. Some girlfriends get messed up because mine are so cute. People know their daddies are nice looking. I obviously have good taste. . . . I just feel as if I'm in more control of things in my life with my family the way it is now.

Because in its romanticized state motherhood represents a social ideal, young women who are seeking respect from their peers and elders may either consciously seek out this status or still passively attain it through, for example, not consistently using contraceptives.

When asked about their expectations of motherhood, five young women emphasized how they thought others would respond to them rather than their personal responsibilities for their children's development. For example, these three alluded to status and image in different ways.

> I always smile at mothers. They just seem settled, you know. I think it will be seen that I am a good person.

> Babies like loving. I will take care of them, always having them wear nice things with their hair done and all.

> As a strong black woman I need to support my community any way I can. My babies are my way of being part of things here.

Teenage females are more aware of what the status of mother represents rather than the set of expectations associated with the role of mother. Young women who do not wish to be parents are more interested in gaining adult status through other markers of achievement, including an advanced education and employment. They clearly articulate the effects the social role and responsibilities associated with motherhood would have on their future. Becoming an adult does not require becoming pregnant.

Sex, Intimacy, and Growing Up

Recognizing the realm in which young women characterize their relationships with men is an essential link to understanding what sex and intimacy mean to them. Intuitively, it is reasonable to argue that young women who seek to pair off with one partner might construct their sexual needs differently from women who are less interested in maintaining one relationship. One possible hypothesis is that young women searching for committed relationships will be inclined to comply with their partners' sexual needs. In contrast, then, teenage women who do not want such relationships will be less responsive to sexual pressure because they are not fearful of losing a potential romantic and intimate partner. An alternate argument is that relationship-oriented young women will be unwilling to engage in sexual activity without a commitment from their partner whereas more sex-oriented teens will do so because they do not wish to lose a potential sexual partner.

According to research on adolescent sexuality, teenagers of all ages and ethnicities are influenced by their perceptions of peer activities and attitudes.[49] Young women with greater internal loci of control (a belief that they can control their own destiny), who often come from higher SES backgrounds, are more likely to equate sex with love than young women from less secure households. Teenagers from economically stable families are also more likely to have two parents or guardians in the household providing them with role models regarding romantic and sexual relationships.[50]

Decisions over the timing of sexual activity are the result of a variety of societal, interpersonal, and individual factors. Young women who consider sex a romantic act of love to be shared with a special partner are more likely to abstain. Those who define sexual activity in terms of the risk of pregnancy and the subsequent change in lifestyle will abstain. In most cases, abstention is associated with the perception of an adult future, one that is defined by more than the ability to have sex and reproduce. Teenagers whose parents have expressed the importance of virginity but who maintain open communication concerning sex are also less likely to initiate sexual activity in their early teens.

Factors associated with an increased chance of early sexual activity are often contradictory. Young women who have few life options and who experience social isolation within their communities are more likely to become sexually active young. Sexual intercourse represents a moment of intimacy and escape from their social situation.[51] These young women do not necessarily trust their sexual partners, nor do they consider their sexual contact an emotional commitment. Many of these young women have had little or no interaction with a respected adult concerning their developing sexuality and are extremely uncomfortable with their sexuality. They report more sex guilt than those who abstain, and they claim to respect young women who are virgins.

Many of these variables are also associated with contraceptive use among the sexually active young women. In the following chapter, the effect of perceived life chances, alienation, intimacy, romantic images of sex, and age on contraceptive decision making will be discussed in detail. All of this provides some insight into the way teenagers rationalize their sexual activity and contraceptive use and what causes risk taking.

6

Contraception:
Safer Sex or Birth Control?

How does someone choose birth control? Anyone who is sexually active or ready to begin sexual activity is faced with a vast array of choices and challenges. First is the question of avoiding pregnancy, and now in this AIDS era, the concern also arises of preventing HIV. Science is constantly investigating new contraceptive methods. In the past few years we have been introduced to Norplant, the sponge (recently removed from the market), and the female condom. Controversy over the availability of RU-486, also known as the "abortion" pill, as well as the lack of new male-focused options rages on. We could argue that at the heart of the debate over birth control are the same questions plaguing the debates over teenage sexuality. We need to recognize that adolescents are sexually active in order to seriously consider their perceptions of the effectiveness and appeal of various contraceptive methods. When compared with adults, teenagers may face qualitatively different kinds of issues when selecting contraception. We need to inquire into the ways the merits of pregnancy prevention are weighed against the merits of STD prevention in order to understand why so few teenagers (and adults) are using condoms regularly.

Central to the debate over sex and AIDS education is contraception. Young men and women are faced with the same choices (including not using contraception) concerning reproduction and protection that adults face. Social and cultural influences on what they know, and how their choices are shaped, remain extensive. In addition to developing relationship skills, teenagers are also coming to grips with a world that is simultaneously ever changing and static. More elements are involved with the decision to use contraception than meet the eye. Furthermore, because so few teenagers using contraception even consider condoms—the only contraceptive that limits the risk of infection—there are apparently key symbolic differences between condom use and other contraceptive choices.

Choosing to contracept (using any form of contraception) is very different from choosing to use condoms. Many young women believe in contracepting but do not include condoms in their range of options. Others, since AIDS became a health concern, have begun to use condoms exclusively. It is possible that what motivates a young woman to consider contraception may not compel her to choose condoms in particular. The teenagers of concern to me, and to those engaged in sex education and AIDS prevention, are the young women whose decision making exposes them to any amount of risk: those using condoms erratically, those using any method but condoms, those using ineffective methods of pregnancy prevention, and, of course, those using no contraception at all.

Contraception prevents pregnancy. The terminology used for these methods—birth control and contraception—makes clear that these were invented during an era when the issue was preventing pregnancy, not preventing the transmission of STDs. Medically approved methods—whether female or male, long term or short term, over the counter or prescribed—prevent conception most of the time when used properly. Because so many different types of contraception are available, young adults have to decide on what form of birth control they will use. Contraceptive methods appeal to young women for different reasons. Comfort, expense, ease of use, popularity, and accessibility are all factored into their decision making.[1] Some methods do have additional purposes, such as the pill, which restricts the growth of fibroids and regulates menstruation. In general, though, pregnancy prevention is the commonly viewed purpose of contraception. We have spent most of this century linking contraception with pregnancy prevention. So, what would cause a young women to think in terms to choose, or reject, condoms?

Deciding whether to use condoms is a complex process. First, a young woman must acquire a certain amount of contraceptive knowledge and also have positive feelings about contracepting. Second, she must want to prevent a pregnancy and believe that she is able to do so. Third, she must want to avoid HIV infection. A few stumbling blocks may stand in the way of choosing condoms. She may not recognize that there is a possible risk of exposure to HIV when not using condoms, or she may assess her chances of contracting HIV inaccurately. She may be so concerned over a partner's response to introducing condoms into the relationship that she talks herself out of even considering condoms.

Also, the need to avoid pregnancy may outweigh her interest in avoiding infection.

Because so much is factored into selecting contraceptives in general, and condoms in particular, one school of thought proposes that anyone deciding on contraception must first go through a number of stages. According to ARRM (AIDS Risk Reduction Model) and the HBM (Health Belief Model), knowing about AIDS and HIV, determining risk, committing to reducing risk, and using the appropriate means will usually result in condom use. Another theory, called rational choice, posits that an individual will consider the varying costs and benefits associated first with contraception then with condom use. One's choice is determined by whichever option offers her more benefits than costs and liabilities. These models, however, do not incorporate some other important factors that appear to influence interest in condom use. The Health Decision Model is similar to the two previous ones, but it also includes attention to more contextual variables:

> [D]ecisions to change health-related attitudes and behaviors are made with some attention to our past experiences with other people who are important to us, our knowledge of others' views and opinions, and our current interactions with others. . . . [W]e need to look at the larger social context in which the person lives. For example, in the case of condom use, we need to consider cultural values related to condoms.[2]

Perceptions of one's social position, relationships with others, receptiveness to others' opinions, and culture are relevant in the contraceptive selection process.

Exclusion from educational and economic opportunity and social isolation resulted in a dearth of resources offering young women accurate information about AIDS prevention. As a result of this, as well as perceptions perpetuated by friends in the community, much of the AIDS folklore circulating among teenagers remained unchallenged. For example, a common assumption among the young women was that you could determine by sight whether a person had HIV. This very popular perception was reinforced because the teenagers did not have alternate sources of information. Second, lack of resources resulted in poor health and medical attention, including family planning and counseling. Furthermore, the constant threat of loss—of friends, relatives, and neighbors—often led to a young woman isolating herself emotionally from others. As a result of infrequent and short-term romantic relationships, these women either mistrust men or will avoid any issues that might cost them a potential relationship. They refuse to address the need to use condoms because this decision first requires emotional intimacy with and trust in one's partner; they do not believe they have the time to develop this sort of bond with their partner. Instead, this emotional connection can be derived quickly through sexual contact.

This constant threat of loss, coupled with irregular employment and absent social support, modifies what risk means. Finding work, protecting oneself from violence, and raising children are more important issues than calculating the probability of contracting an STD. The prevailing attitude is that risking the loss of a sexual partner through introducing the issue of AIDS into a relationship is greater than the inevitable loss of life. Death is inevitable. Finally, condoms no longer represent contraception—they symbolize disease prevention. The negative impact of introducing condoms into a relationship is multiplied as a result.

The cultural and social symbolism in condom use is of utmost importance in the decision-making process. A teenage woman's emotional bond with her partner and feelings of trust in him influence condom use. What condoms, personal risk, and AIDS *mean* has to be understood before condom use will increase among teenage women of color.

Using Contraceptives

Considering that rates of teenage pregnancy and STD infection remain high, it is apparent that not enough young adults are using effective contraceptive methods regularly. Younger sexually active teenagers are the ones least likely to consider birth control as a realistic and necessary presence in their sexual lives.[3] In one study, only one-third of all black teenagers regularly used an effective means of contraception, and of this group, 68 percent never used condoms.[4] In their landmark study on sex and pregnancy, Melvin Zelnik, John Kantner, and Kathleen Ford (1981) considered the effects of age, race, family background, and religion on the contraceptive choices of young women in 1971 and 1976.[5] A main assumption was that young women who reported using contraception both the first and last times they had sexual intercourse were probably using contraception regularly. The researchers made this assumption because using contraceptives the first time one has sex is uncommon; such a young woman is probably more willing to anticipate any sexual activity and actually to plan on using contraceptives.

According to their data, about 60 percent of the young women who had sex did not use any form of contraception during their first sexual experience. The researchers noted a slight difference between white and black respondents. Forty percent of white teens between fifteen and nineteen used some contraceptive method, whereas about one-third of black teens used contraception. There were greater racial differences in terms of the kind of contraceptive used. Over 40 percent of contracepting black teens used the pill, diaphragm, or IUD, whereas only one-fifth of whites relied on these methods. What this means is that white teenagers probably used condoms more than other methods.

Zelnik et al. argue that using a medical method indicates a willingness to prepare for sexual activity in advance because medical contraceptives require examinations and prescriptions.[6] Theoretically, for a proactive teenager, sexual activity cannot be completely spontaneous if one plans on using a medical method—this is especially true for diaphragms, which have to be fitted by a doctor, must be applied before intercourse, and thus can interfere with spontaneity.[7] One conclusion is that because they use medical methods so often, black teenagers in their sample were more willing to prepare before having sex. However, advance planning does not guarantee contraceptives will actually be used during sex. Given the irregularity of contraceptive use among black teenage girls in the study, preparation did not translate into regular usage. Studies that indicate that young black women are more willing to consider using contraception before engaging in sex may conclude that black women are more committed to protection. But we need to remember that on the whole they are also more erratic in contraceptive use.

By 1982, according to a study sponsored by the Alan Guttmacher Institute, the numbers of never-married young women who used contraceptives at least once increased to almost three out of four.[8] Unfortunately, only 34 percent of these respondents used contraception consistently. The young women used birth control during their last sexual experience but not when they initiated sexual activity:

Forty-five percent of women aged 15–19 in 1979 who were premaritally sexually active and who did not practice contraception at first intercourse started doing so subsequently. Seventy percent . . . interviewed in 1979 reported that they had used a contraceptive method the last time they had intercourse, an increase of 19 percentage points since the first time they had intercourse. . . . Sixty-nine percent . . . aged 15–19 in 1982 who had had intercourse within the previous three months and were not pregnant, postpartum, or seeking pregnancy had practiced contraception during the previous month. Sixty-two percent of these women had used the pill.[9]

Since the emergence of HIV and AIDS in the early to mid-1980s, the proportion of young women using condoms has increased markedly. George Lowenstein and Frank Furstenberg (1991) report an increase in the number of young women using birth control at last intercourse.[10] Black women reported the lowest rate of birth control usage at first intercourse (37 percent), but during their last sexual encounter they surpass Latinas in usage. Overall, the risk of pregnancy and STD infection was greater among some blacks because of greater sexual activity, earlier initiation of sex, and less reliance on protection.

Contraceptive Options: Who Contracepts?

Facing the prospect of using birth control is both exciting and intimidating considering the vast array of options available. What may be unsurprising is that the young woman who investigates and actively chooses to use contraception may be the same woman who delays having intercourse until her late teens. A young woman who actively contemplates and considers her sexual options is displaying the kinds of skills found in young women who use contraception regularly. Teenage girls who have sex at a young age but still manage to use birth control appear to have personalities and family histories that are similar to those of young women who delay or abstain from sex altogether. For example, there is a connection between economic background—social class—and both the age a young woman first has sex and contraceptive use. Young women who live with both parents and whose mothers have at least twelve years of education are likely to use some method.

> The mother's level of education represents the socio-economic level of the family; it may also tap the aspirations of the young woman for what Hogan and Kitagawa called a "path to adulthood," in which childbearing is delayed until after a woman's education is completed and she obtains a good job. If the woman sees these goals as the only acceptable way to attain adult status, early parenthood becomes unacceptable and contraceptive use during premarital intercourse is more likely.[11]

Those who delayed engaging in intercourse until they were at least sixteen will probably use contraception from the onset of activity.[12]

Young women who learn about sex and contraception while young and are taught to be comfortable with their sexuality will probably use contraceptives correctly and consistently. Comfort with talking about sexuality and pregnancy is also associated with using contraception all of the time. The messages communicated when parents educated young girls about sex appeared to affect how these young girls would eventually behave. The teenage girls who engage in early, unprotected sex were often from socially and economically compromised communities. This view was confirmed by the observations of some poor teens. The meaning of sex and the need to maintain emotional separation from one's partners were directly connected with condom use.

The young woman who has learned little about sex at an older age than women from socially and economically mainstream families is likely to believe she cannot and should not maintain control over her sexual choices. She frequently experiences a great deal of guilt concerning her sexual activity. A young woman experiencing these emotions will wish to avoid any reminders that she is doing something as "bad" as having sex. Naturally, even the thought of birth control is too much of a reminder, and it challenges her presumption that her sexual life is out of her hands. She is therefore at a great risk for not contracepting, especially with condoms. This is clearly operating in a comment made by one teenager, Nina, from a low-income family. Not discussing sex and contraception resulted in Nina guessing about the timing of her ovulating.

> I can tell you when I could become pregnant because I can feel it in my body. At those times I just avoid sleeping with a guy. . . . My mom didn't exactly sit me down to talk about it. . . . You know, it's something you just take care of when you can, without letting people get in your business.

For Nina, planning and using contraceptives required recognizing her sexual activity. As her mother had taught her, sex was to be kept secret. The less one knew about it, the better. This is one situation in which lacking information, not assuming active control over one's sexuality, and feeling sex guilt resulted in risky contraceptive behavior.

Marsha's beliefs about contraceptive behavior are different. She grew up in an economically diverse neighborhood, and her family was middle class. She learned about sex young but did not know about contraception until she was much older. Even so, she felt comfortable choosing contraception because of her comfort with her sexuality. Marsha made contraceptive choices that involved planning and information gathering.

> When I started talking with Walter, I kind of liked him. So we were talking for a while when we started. . . . I thought we could have sex, so I made sure we had condoms all of the time just in case. . . . I didn't want to be without one when it happened. . . . He had some also. . . . When we went together a while I went to the [health] center to see a doctor about

maybe getting the pill too. I knew it would make pregnancy less possible.
. . . Using both makes me feel I'm really safer.

Marsha was more proactive than Nina by planning her sexual activity, seeking out and using contraception.

Though the rates of contraceptive use have increased among black teenagers over the last fifteen years, most still do not use condoms regularly. Surveys of seventh and eighth graders indicate that males were more comfortable with male methods (i.e., condoms and withdrawal) and females preferred the pill and the sponge—female methods.[13] This finding points to the powerful influence socially determined gender norms and expectations have on attitudes. Comfort with contraceptive use was associated with methods the respondents could control, but these adolescents still believed that reproductive and contraceptive responsibility (procuring and using them) should fall to young women; both sexes believed that females should be responsible for contraception because they were the ones who faced the risk of pregnancy. Of course, responsibility falls on both partners' shoulders, but the popular social norm is that women are responsible for anything associated with bearing and raising children. Many young men expect young women to be sexually progressive but socially traditional. Feminist scholars have noted this "madonna–whore" conflict: be enticing and sexually available but also be "the kind of girl one can bring home to mother."[14]

Contraceptive Options: Who Uses Condoms?

The increase in birth control use is heartening, but too few people are tested for AIDS and/or use condoms. Teenagers are still very resistant to the idea that it is important to consider changing sexual behaviors such as many sexual partners and unprotected vaginal, anal, and oral-genital contact. Current findings regarding condom use are misleading. Even though recent studies have recorded marked increases in condom use, questions still surround the frequency and regularity of this use. Additionally, those using condoms are still in the minority. In one study of 1,244 teenage women fifteen to nineteen years old, the number of teens using condoms doubled between 1979 and 1988.[15] According to their findings, more black teens used condoms than whites. The proportion of blacks reporting use had almost tripled since 1979 (from 23.2 percent to 62 percent). Over half of white, black, and Latino teens used condoms as opposed to 21 percent in 1979. Unfortunately, one out of every five used an ineffective contraceptive method (e.g., withdrawal or the rhythm method) at last intercourse.

What has happened since more people have become aware of the threat of HIV infection and AIDS? Has there been a substantial shift in condom use? More recent data on AIDS-related behavior show that 15 percent of unmarried teenage girls who were sexually active in the month prior to being surveyed report always using condoms. The percentage reporting having ever used latex condoms during intercourse was about half of all sexually active teenage girls.[16] Only 9 percent changed at least one risky behavior and used condoms.[17] When race is factored in, a few distinctions emerge. Among non-Latino blacks, 15 percent always use condoms, 40 percent occasionally use condoms or have changed their sexual behavior, and 7 percent changed behavior and use condoms. Eighteen percent of non-Latino whites always use condoms, 53 percent use condoms or have changed behavior, and 12 percent use condoms and have changed behaviors. Data from another study show less marked changes in condom use for blacks.[18]

What these studies indicate is that although more black teenage girls are actively using contraception (even if the consistency of use is unclear), there are contradictions concerning condom use. This observation is problematic when considered in the social context in which teenagers address the threats of AIDS and HIV infection. Teenagers continue to focus on pregnancy prevention when choosing contraception, not disease prevention. At the same time, they are very aware that symbolically condoms are associated with STDs. They consider all of this information when trying to determine whether they personally are at risk for pregnancy and STDs. Often teenagers may conclude that condoms are not always necessary. In fact, I came to realize that some used condoms only if they were deemed absolutely necessary. What "absolutely necessary" meant varied with the specific circumstances young women experienced. For some, condoms were only absolutely necessary with a stranger, not with a boyfriend who "played around." For others, condoms were absolutely necessary when they were menstruating. Because of these various distinctions, it is apparent that teenagers may report using condoms regularly, but for them, regularity was conditional—only when absolutely necessary.

How Regular Is Condom Use?

Among the sexually active women I met, a slight majority reported condom use. More than half of them stated that they had used condoms during sexual activity in the past year. This includes young women who use them regularly as well as those who use them sporadically. One third of all the teenagers who reported condom use did so often but not always. Some of the participants claimed to use condoms more than they actually did. In these cases, contradictory information from our discussions is what enabled me to question their reported usage. For example, Sara was describing a number of instances in which the condom had broken during intercourse.

> **Sara:** I'm tired of these sorry rubbers not working. I spend half of my time worrying about them being good or bad brands. Sometimes free ones are all dried out, so they don't work.
> **RTW:** What do you do, then, when they are dried out?
> **Sara:** I get pissed because you're already into things. Who'd ever think of doing a test run with a condom before talking to a guy? . . . So I usually try to get out of it.
> **RTW:** Out of . . .
> **Sara:** Out of the sex.
> **RTW:** But how do you do that, I mean isn't it . . .
> **Sara:** Yes. Oh, what did you say? [inaudible] Oh, I try to slow things down, but you know how men get when they're ready and good to go on. . . . So I slow him down.
> **RTW:** Okay, I see what you mean there, but what do you do without a condom?
> **Sara:** Oh, I stall for time and maybe go through with it if he's okay.
> **RTW:** What makes him okay?
> **Sara:** He's pretty clean, and we are friendly enough. And if I really am in the mood, then maybe we'll still do it without a rubber. But I don't get too into it, because we aren't using one.

In another instance, a young woman who stated that she and her boyfriend only have sex with a condom ended up contradicting this claim a number of times:

> He really hates them but uses them because I want to. Once when we were messing around he asked about how it felt without one, if I'd think about trying it. We did, *just once,* and that was it. That was the one time it happened.

In response to a question about planning how many condoms she usually had available, she said:

> Well, he never has them, since he doesn't believe in condoms. He figures I should get them. . . . I never know how many I should carry with me. If I run out before I get to Planned Parenthood, I deal. . . . Once we used a sponge, but I thought it was awful. It smelled funny.

This young woman has confused her contraceptive use with the frequency of condom use. In recording frequency of use, then, studies have to clearly define what that means.

Studying contraceptive use commonly involves interview or survey items that range from "always/regularly use" to "never use."[19] However, what many conversations highlighted was that teenagers (and most likely adults as well) were imprecise when reporting frequency of their own condom use.

Aside from the risk of pregnancy, erratic condom use is playing Russian roulette with HIV infection. In the cases in which use was not accurately reported, young women tended to define frequent use with consistent use. As the preceding quotations show, "almost always" using a condom could quickly turn into "always." In assessing one's risk, these kind of allowances are problematic. A second category of women, who use condoms with men they believe are risky partners, also call their condom use regular. This is because they are using them on a regular basis with one category of men. These women do not believe they have to use a condom with "safe" men. Of course, this argument means that on occasion they are relying on visual and other cues to define a safe partner and are still exposing themselves to possible infection.

Condom Use: Fear of Infection, Fear of Pregnancy

There is a difference between deciding to use any form of contraception and wanting to make that option condoms. The motivation to contracept is a necessary, but not sufficient, precursor to condom use. To make the shift from committing to contracept to using only condoms, one has to believe in the effectiveness of condoms and be concerned about HIV infection.

Apart from education about AIDS, this point implies that teenagers have to be at least as concerned about the risk of sexually transmitted diseases as they are about the risk of becoming pregnant.[20] As Susie asserts, "no girl should be without [condoms]. What's the reason in avoiding a pregnancy if you could still get something and maybe even die? What would you have then? . . . My folks gave me more sense than that." If a teenager is not concerned about HIV infection and believes that they minimize pleasure and require interrupting intercourse, then she is likely to consider other methods or nothing at all. "Condoms get in the way during sex," said Evelyn. "It makes sex feel strange. I want to feel close to my man." Even though free condoms are available from many clinics and organizations, most teens still do not use them consistently.

Even though more black teens have reported using condoms, only a small percentage use them regularly. Most of those who are regular users were from middle-class or upper-middle-class families. Regardless of race, those using condoms are committed to their partners' well-being, accept themselves as sexual people, have exchanged information about sex with parents and friends, and have a defined and positive future outlook.[21]

Relative Meanings of Risk

Deciding to use condoms is dependent on an accurate assessment of risk, a willingness to obtain condoms, and a positive view of condoms.[22] Both risk assessment and a willingness to obtain information about condoms are products of a decision-making process occurring in the stages outlined by the Health Belief and AIDS Risk Reduction Models.[23] An understanding of the causes of HIV infection and AIDS, as well as faith in the usefulness of condoms, does not always translate into risk reduction. An individual must accurately assess her own risk of infection. Sherry, at seventeen, has received sex education in her high school and "the minimal birds and bees stuff" from her parents. Though active with more than one sexual partner, she has never used condoms. She has been tested for HIV twice and appears to believe that these negative results are proof that condoms are unnecessary.

Sherry: I've had sex for long enough that if I were getting HIV I would have it by now. I believe that because the guys I am with aren't into anything too strange, I am not in danger. I've even been pregnant before, so shouldn't that mean I cannot get AIDS at this time?

RTW: Why did you get tested if you don't consider yourself at risk for HIV infection?

Sherry: Because I did want to make sure. Not all of the guys in my past were great. Some probably did get themselves into trouble. You know.

RTW: Like what kind of trouble?

Sherry: Using the pipe, snorting.

RTW: So do drugs make someone at risk?

Sherry: Yeah.

RTW: Anything else?

Sherry: Kinky, weird sex and stuff. Homo stuff. Getting it off the streets.

RTW: What about having sex with lots of different people? A lot of doctors and experts believe that every time you have sex with someone, you are also sleeping with everyone that they've slept with. Have you heard about that?

Sherry: Yes. I bet a lot of people should deal with that. . . . [I'm] lucky because I only hang around with guys I know, and they aren't with a lot of other girls either.

Sherry's definition of risk is different from standard public health guidelines. Traditionally, multiple sexual partners, substance use (or sexual contact with an injection drug user), and unprotected contact with one's partner all qualify as high-risk activities. Her sense of personal responsibility extends only as far as taking an AIDS test. Even if her information base is not completely accurate, she does have a sense of what constitutes risky behavior. However, she does not include her behavior in that category.

Unless a young woman accurately defines risk in terms of behaviors that result in infection, no amount of knowledge will result in using condoms or otherwise reducing risk: "Efforts to prevent disease are motivated primarily by actual risk of disease."[24] Believing that one is at risk is directly shaped by the social reality a women faces; a young woman will assess her own risk, as well as the risk posed by others, in the context of her everyday life. Both what a young woman defines as risky behavior and the potential impact that risk may have on her are judgments influenced by more than access to information.

For example, family and peers affect how a young woman defines risky behavior in general as well as her own personal risk. Perceptions of present opportunity are clearly associated with young women's views of their future and subsequently how they act in shaping their future. These assessments are emotional and visceral; this is not necessarily an instance in which one consciously plans to behave in a particular way. Consider, for example, young women who accidentally become pregnant; they face a permanent change in their lives as well as the possibility of HIV infection. When asked why they got pregnant, a common response was that "it just happened." Such a response is frequently perceived as evidence that teenagers do not think about the consequences of their actions. In fact, what might have happened is something very different. If motherhood represents a potential increase in respect and status, these teenagers may be less inclined to see pregnancy as a problem or a threat to avoid. This view would be particularly relevant for young women who have few opportunities to attain those trappings associated with adulthood. As one stated succinctly, "I'm grown now that I have a baby. No more playing." Motherhood becomes appealing if it is one of the few social statuses a young woman believes she can achieve. Without a change in the social and economic environment, there will be few motives for using any form of contraception, let alone condoms.

Young women who believe their environment offers opportunity for growth and advancement will actively prevent pregnancy, and probably HIV infection, because they believe they can and will become successful adults. For Jane, the thought of having a child during adolescence "makes no sense since I have stuff to do. I want to be a mom in the future, but I have to get myself on track. Right now I'm too young for that responsibility." The overwhelming majority of young women I met who were not pregnant (by choice) perceived other social opportunities that were more important than motherhood. They had a vision of the future where finishing high school, finding work, and attending college predated pregnancy. One of the strongest examples was Chris, who avoided not only sexual activity but also drug and alcohol use because they could "lead to something more than what [she was] ready for." A person considers the life she presently has and decides on the kinds of future she may have. She then may behave in ways that are based on such social realities.

Interactions with friends and family, and in the community, provide young women with the social context through which their identities are codified. This sense of self is what determines how young women perceive their future options. For middle-class teens the future is filled with opportunities—they have choices. As Linda reports, when she and her friends talk about the future, she sees a place for family life: "I'm young. Things can still happen. I want to be with kids and a husband. . . . My girlfriends and I talk about what things will be like in a few years, with kids, men, and such. . . . We have plans." Marian is also preparing for the future:

> So I know most people will stay in this town, maybe finishing school, maybe getting a regular paycheck. . . . I want to set up in Atlanta where my brother and cousin are. . . . right here my first plan is to work and get money to move. Kevin [her son] and I will move on soon.

Each of these young women clearly articulates how her relationships both shaped and reinforced her future plans. Perceptions of the future mediate behavior.

Recognizing opportunities, and being able to remain optimistic about the future, influenced the expectations they had for themselves and their friends. Setting boundaries on behavior became important. As Linda explained,

> So I'll go to school, probably Southern [Connecticut State University] or UNH [University of New Haven]. . . . That is primary for now. . . . Some

things can wait until later. If people don't want to handle that, they can step off. People will come and go.

Marian described meeting someone who could have convinced her to postpone or give up her plans:

> I met someone who was good, or so I thought. He turned out to be not serious and just partied. We were good together, but that won't give my baby a future. He kept coming by and staying over. That was fine until I saw that he wasn't going anywhere . . . basically doing nothing. I'm not taking that to Atlanta.

What is fascinating is that in both situations the young woman focuses on the barriers to her future opportunity. Risky behavior then becomes defined as anything that would interfere with the realization of this goal. Risky behavior is not defined specifically as actions leading to contracting an STD or becoming pregnant. This is a subtle, yet important distinction. If someone, or something, might interfere with the plans a young woman has made for herself, then she is motivated to avoid him, her, or it. Contracting HIV and becoming pregnant were not seen as risks and problems in their own right.

Many times teenagers may be able to define risk accurately, and to some extent "personalize" it, without initiating condom use or minimizing other behaviors associated with HIV infection.[25] Sexually active young women accurately identify multiple sex partners, intravenous drug use, not using condoms, and sex with and HIV positive partner as risky activities. While many describe behaving in ways that clearly placed them at high risk, few actually acknowledge that they were in fact at-risk. Three girls describe their assessment of risk:

> Yes, I've been tested for HIV. They've come out negative (thank God). Just because the guys I was really, really sexually active with in the last four years or so ran a high chance of being HIV + . After learning more about HIV, I had to make sure I wasn't positive of HIV. I believe I was very lucky of the fact that I was never infected with any kind of infections or diseases and that I was never, ever pregnant in my life, yet. Before I didn't know and I didn't care and I didn't worry. Now, I know, I care, and I do worry. Sometimes too much. I'm actually considering not having sex until I get married.[26]

> There's no way I could get AIDS because my boyfriend and I are only with each other. I don't like condoms and he doesn't either so we don't use them. I get a sponge from the store every once in a while because I do not want any babies yet. . . . I never been with anyone before Carl, but

he had girlfriends. I hear one says he got her pregnant, but I don't believe it. He wouldn't do that.

Some weekends the party scene is real good, other times not. A little to drink is always a party, loosens folk up; they get stupid. I have met a few guys at parties and hooked up with them. I probably will be sorry that I don't use condoms at all, and I probably should start now, but I only have sex once, then it isn't a big deal.[27]

According to the Health Belief Model and the AIDS Risk Reduction Model, accurately identifying one's personal vulnerability to HIV and expressing a willingness to change behavior must precede lasting and effective behavior change such as using condoms all of the time.[28] Rational choice/contraceptive decision-making theory has also established that an individual will avoid risking infection or pregnancy because she believes in using condoms and wishes to avoid or at least minimize her risk of pregnancy. Because the majority of those using contraceptives do not use protection regularly and rarely use condoms, it is apparent that these youth are not fulfilling at least one of these prerequisites.

Condom Use: Emotional and Symbolic Influences

Young women who accurately perceive their susceptibility or risk of AIDS and STD infection or pregnancy are more willing to use condoms exclusively than ones who have a false sense of security. Girls who know a great deal still misinterpret their own personal risk of infection. Consequently, they may be unwilling to change their behavior in order to lower their risk. Young women in monogamous relationships, with few lifetime sexual partners, who do not identify themselves as risk takers often inaccurately assess their relative risk. They are less willing to change their sexual or contraceptive behavior to minimize the risk of infection.[29] A younger teenager who expresses high levels of guilt about her sexuality, has negative views of sexuality, and infrequently has sex will probably avoid using condoms.[30] Older teenage women have sex more regularly than younger ones and report using condoms more than younger teens.[31] What emerges from these findings is that older, sexually active teens are more comfortable with their sexuality and with discussions about condom use with their partner(s).

Wanting to rely on medical methods such as the pill and diaphragm is dependent on something frequently expressed by the teenagers—a need for independence and autonomy in one's sex life. In the previous chapter I illustrated how fear of intimacy and lack of trust resulted in many participants not wanting emotional involvement with their partners. Condom use requires at least the involvement and consent of the male partner. Some equate this involvement with a dependence on men; it follows that teens who distrust men might wish to avoid this kind of dependence on their partner. In contrast, those who depend on men for validation may be swayed by their partner's opinion of condoms.

What will enable a young woman, in spite of these attitudes, to use condoms and to use them consistently? Dooley Worth[32] illustrates why black young women who are active and comfortable with their sexuality are unwilling to use condoms. Younger teenagers, who have learned to meet their partners' needs at any cost, are taught to depend on men for sexual validation. They learn that a man's desires supersede theirs. The shortage of black men in more socially isolated urban communities can result in truncated relationships—interactions in which both partners do not jointly decide to sever sexual contact. A young woman is less likely to insist on having her needs met, whether sexual or otherwise, because it might result in his severing their relationship.[33] Worth contends, "Culturally determined values influence how individual perceptions of AIDS are selected, how attitudes toward high-risk behavior are formed, how habits that characterize high-risk behavior are developed, and how risk-reduction information will be processed."[34]

For young women who are concerned about maintaining relationships, the potential repercussions of losing a romantic partner are more frightening than the potential risk of pregnancy and contracting an STD. Instead, various contradictions exist. Young women are assessing their relative risks inaccurately, though they are aware of how risky behavior is defined. They strongly believe in contraceptive use but not necessarily condom use. The same young women I met who spoke proudly of being in control were at the same time less likely to use any birth control.

Older teenagers with a great deal of sexual experience were comfortable with their sexuality and claimed responsibility for their sexual activity. Most of these women were also pregnant or already had children. They considered the role of a man in their lives as mainly sexual. Any emotional involvement would be an unexpected bonus. Because emotional contact and intimacy were not expected, they were unwilling to "waste" time talking about condoms because, as one woman claimed, "men can't be trusted any further than the length of their dicks." These perceptions are surprising because we often assume women who consider themselves responsible for their own sexuality would also consider condom use part of this responsibility for them-selves.

What Condoms Represent

Additional factors influencing condom use are the social values attached to condoms and to using them. Because of the social "value" or popular perception of condoms, teenagers who can accurately as-sess their own risk of exposure to HIV may still avoid contracepting with condoms. All teenagers are privy to such social definitions, which makes it even more difficult to determine whether social class and fam-ily stability affect one's perception of risk and of condoms. Contrary to conventional wisdom, contraceptive responsibility is not simply de-pendent on social class position. Middle-class teenagers who are well informed may not use condoms because of what condoms symbolize for them.

One such middle-class girl, fifteen years old and sexually active for three years, believed that all contraceptive planning is "bad news, be-cause people will think you are sleeping around and that you do it with anything." Here the social value placed on sexual purity (at least the appearance of purity) increased her worry that condom use will call her purity into question. For her, and other sexually active young women I spoke with, contraceptives would ruin either their or their partner's reputation.

A variety of explanations underlie this argument. First, any advance planning might ruin the "fun and surprise of just being with some-one." Second, the opinion that birth control is expensive, cumbersome, and hard to obtain prevails to a great extent. Finally, a few teenagers believe that "only older kids can get pregnant and stuff. [We] don't have to get into that for a few years." When I asked this fifteen-year-old whether she had ever met a girl under sixteen who was pregnant or already had a child, she told me, "Yeah, but she must not have done it right, 'cause if she had, she wouldn't have been having a baby."

These comments highlight some of the social-psychological are asso-ciated with birth control use. Underlying beliefs in the usefulness of contraception (physiological—as a barrier to pregnancy and STDs—and social—as a symbol of one's reputation), combined with percep-tions of potential risks associated with not using contraception, deter-mine whether a teenager will even consider birth control an option. Though teens are generally aware of contraceptive options, they are less aware of (or concerned with) pregnancy and the consequences of teen parenthood.[35]

Condoms are commonly associated with disease prevention. Although they also offer protection from pregnancy, sexually active teens minimize this purpose and mainly focus on disease.[36] Most contraceptive information has traditionally focused on pregnancy prevention, not STD avoidance, so teenagers tend to be more receptive to the idea of not getting pregnant than they are to the idea of not contracting HIV. Because teenagers generally underestimate their risk of infection, their resistance to the message to use condoms is not surprising. In one study, 71 percent of black teenage respondents believed that condoms were "too much trouble," and 83 percent felt AIDS was so uncommon that they did not need to worry about infection.[37]

Among poor teenagers of color, another opinion also affects the regularity of use. Desensitization to loss and death weaken the impact a prevention message can have on them.[38] Costs and benefits assigned to using condoms in particular have less meaning. Without the promise of social mobility and in a social setting where other teenagers die regularly, risk reduction is often meaningless.[39] DaNeesha lives with older cousins and very calmly explained that mortality had little meaning to her.

> Last night I was sitting on my bed and I see _____ from the window. He was hanging by himself. Then this person pulls something from the other street and walks up to him and points it at his head and "pop, pop, pop" then _____ falls down and his brains are all over the ground and he jumps around for a little while. I guess he is dead. I get on my bed and go to sleep. Who knows who is next. Could be me or you. Many people I know will be gone soon. That's how it is.

While this story is a more extreme and dramatic example, it draws attention to the ways environment and community can actually determine what relative value is placed on the present and future.

Condoms are presented as a means of preventing infections that can ultimately result in death or a diminished quality of life. For this image to be effective, a teenager has to believe that her life is valuable and that it will result in a future of some opportunity. Without a sense of the value of their lives, teenagers may opt to avoid condoms, which are considered clumsy and uncomfortable, or all contraceptives. Condom use is "more likely as the sense of individual vulnerability increases concurrent with the belief that the adverse outcome (AIDS) can be avoided at not too great a cost (decreased sexual pleasure). . . . [We need] to determine what raises the adolescent's sense of vulnerability sufficiently to result in behavioral change."[40]

Marlene, a seventeen-year-old senior, is very different from DaNeesha. She has been sexually active for approximately one year with her boyfriend. She considers their relationship exclusive and committed and strongly believes her partner Shaun has not engaged in any risky behaviors. Even so, she says they always use condoms.

> You got to use at least rubbers these days. I love Shaun, but he knows that if he don't want to do it with them, he's out the door. That saying "no cover, no lover" is how I believe. What's the point of some fun if it means a lot of pain down the line? Sex is great, but life is better. Girls should remember that.

This conversation followed the announcement that Magic Johnson was HIV positive. In previous discussions Marlene had admitted that at times she had considered not using condoms, "to see what it would be like." However, her main worry was that she may contract something or pass a "yeast-like infection or something nasty like that" to him.

Teenagers in monogamous relationships are less willing to introduce condoms into their intimate contacts because they believe that they are not at risk of infection. Sexually active youth who are not in intimate and monogamous relationships do not use condoms because they require input from the partner. Because so many older teens distrust men, they are unwilling to rely on them for disease prevention. Instead, they believe that they can visually determine who is at risk and that other behavioral adjustments can satisfactorily replace relying on condoms.

Addressing Ambivalence about Condoms

Sexuality and contraceptive use are shaped by many elements in young women's lives. Gender and sex roles are learned in households and schools. Peers and the media also provide role models and either reinforce or challenge previously held attitudes and behaviors. Although most young women report experiencing some peer pressure to become sexually active, or at least to appear sexually knowledgeable, not all have been affected by others' expectations. Family dictates concerning acceptable and unacceptable behavior can temper their choices, as do perceptions of other teenagers' behavior.

Reproduction and contraceptive decision making are mediated by issues of control and identity. These issues are especially acute among teenagers. Poor and working poor women are more likely to represent their sexual activity and identity as symbolic of their independence and self-sufficiency. At the same time, their early sexual activity is characterized as a response to boredom, as a need for companionship in a period of social isolation and alienation, and as proof of woman-hood. Having a man equals femininity and womanhood. Being an adult brings with it a level of freedom and choice otherwise absent in their lives.

Not all poor women become active at a young age, nor do all risk HIV infection by using condoms erratically. Those who do not echo a commitment to their future and expect to leave their neighborhoods in search of, as one explained, "something better, something more than what I see here." What all who consistently use condoms share is a strong belief in their self-importance and a belief that their lives can be affected by personal choice.[41] Is it possible that poor black teenage women who are socially isolated and experience a great deal of sexism and racism concerning female sexuality (e.g., women with sexual experience who take control of their sexual lives are derogated, and people of color are *unnaturally* sexual) can fight to control and enjoy their sexuality?

Contraception has value judgments attached to it, just as sexuality and sexual behavior do. Deciding whether to contracept and then which method to use involves weighing the costs and benefits of use and the relative risks involved with each choice and outcome. Of those who use some form of effective protection (which excludes withdrawal and the rhythm method), a minority report consistent use. These few who use contraceptives regularly do so because they simply do not want to risk pregnancy and/or infection. Either of these outcomes and additional repercussions are unacceptable. Whether they have engaged in risky behaviors or not, these young women consider the potential risk more problematic than the benefits of not using protection.

Condoms have practical and symbolic meaning. For the majority who either never contracept with condoms or do it irregularly, the symbolism associated with use is prohibitive. Either the practical outcomes of use are unimportant, or the symbolic meaning of using them is too important. Preventing pregnancy and STD infection are only meaningful and important if the young woman considers these potential outcomes possible. Risk means different things in different situations. Within each situation, the way risk is defined will result in what may sometimes appear to be contradictory, and ineffective, actions.

Condom use requires that a teenager is willing to admit to her sexual activity and that she is comfortable articulating her sexuality with others. Feeling able to control her own life and believing that she is responsible for her behavior increase the chance that a teenager will use condoms. However, planning on and acquiring condoms also necessitates premeditation. She has to plan to have sex, acquire the contraception (perhaps even consult with a health care provider), introduce its use to her partner, and then actually use it. If she already feels some guilt about her sexuality, she may not want to admit that she needs or wants birth control because she appears too experienced. Additionally, she may fear that her partner will believe either she has already contracted a disease or that he may infect her. This concern raises issues of trust and control. How, then, do these matters influence the likelihood a teenager will use condoms?

Issues of control and identity are integral to a young woman's sexuality. For poor teenage women, their sexual activity represents their independence and self-sufficiency. At the same time, their early sexual activity may be an antidote to boredom, the need for companionship in a period of social isolation and alienation, and is proof of womanhood in a context in which few alternate routes (i.e., through employment and material goods) exist. The validation one may receive by having sex is more valuable than the benefits of either abstinence or condom use. The choice not to contracept has immediate results—physical companionship. The choice to contracept and improve her life options will mean little if a young woman's social network and her community cannot offer her a future in which opportunities and choices are available.

There are contradictions posed by what condoms represent. Teenagers realize that condoms represent disease prevention. Though condoms prevent infection, a more overpowering meaning has been attached to them. Introducing condoms is an accusation; one's partner is guilty of either having had unsafe sex, or being diseased. There is concern that the same assumption might be made regarding the young woman considering using condoms in her relationships. Perhaps her partner might think the same of her. As condoms continue to be associated with AIDS, a young woman is less likely to want to use them. Even if the effectiveness of pregnancy prevention were emphasized, the affiliation with disease would remain. Furthermore, many other methods are available that deal with contraception without raising the issue of disease.

Condoms are also associated with intimacy. In counseling and media presentations, condom use is connected to trust and self-respect. However, considering the disease paradigm, condoms actually represent mistrust and dishonesty. For a younger teenager in close relationships, the message of mistrust persuades her to minimize her own risk in order to protect her relationship from the specter of disease inherent in condom use.

Additionally, older teens, especially ones who are alienated/socially isolated, express less faith in men. They are *more* likely to consider condoms because they do not trust in their partner's sexual commitment to them. However, condoms require the partner's involvement. This kind of intimacy is seen as a relinquishing of a woman's power over her sexuality. Having to have a conversation about sexuality, sexual histories, and contraceptive preferences involves a level of emotional connection that they cannot risk.

Thus, teenagers face a series of conflicts that explain why many are not aggressive in using condoms. Those young women who are most likely to consider condoms are also most likely to abstain until their late adolescence and to define self-control and intimacy in different terms. For them, the presence or absence of a sexual partner is not closely tied to their well-being. They believe other opportunities, outside their immediate peer group, define them as independent and successful women.

Discovering such distinctions in perceptions and behavior requires asking teenagers pointed questions about their past relationships. Particularly in considering teenage sexual attitudes and behavior, there is discomfort with characterizing sexually active youth as having the potential to be responsible sexual actors.[42] Though many young women do not contracept or do so irregularly, many adults over twenty-one also engage in highly risky behavior.[43] Nonetheless, we are less likely to label sexually active adults as irresponsible. Understanding contraceptive use and sexual activity among teenagers also involves a willingness to identify them first as sexual beings, not simply as being sexually compulsive.

7

Ultimate Risk:
Perceptions of AIDS and HIV

The future of too many young adults in the United States will depend on their ability to avoid contracting HIV. As noted by the Office of National AIDS Policy in *Youth and HIV/AIDS: An American Agenda* (1996) "Adolescents need the tools to successfully navigate an increasingly dangerous world. . . . They must be shown the dangers they may encounter and taught negotiation and decision-making skills. . . . And they need to exert personal responsibility to protect both themselves and other from infection."[1] What must they be taught and by whom? At one time educators and public health experts claimed that information and knowledge would arm teenagers with the tools necessary to protect themselves. Teaching was the route to long-lasting and effective risk reduction. Young men and women have the knowledge, but do they have the tools and the faith in the importance of behavior change? Do they believe that they should live their lives differently?

Literature on AIDS education and health initiatives exists in great numbers. Some focuses on the content of programs, others deal with the effectiveness of programs, while still others address the retention of knowledge among program participants. In all three cases, a fundamental issue remains; what do teenagers do with this knowledge? Among the issues of interest is not only where and how young black women learn about HIV and AIDS but whether this information effectively influences behavior change. My intent here is to use the information presented in previous chapters to provide an overview of the ways teenagers are learning about HIV and sex. The implications in these chapters is that the development of sexual identity, the social meaning of sex, adulthood, and motherhood, along with the relative influence of AIDS and risk in their lives, all provide guidelines for educational programs and interventions. Furthermore, I will consider how they perceive the information presented to them and the ways they incorporate the information into their daily lives. What young women have shared with me illuminates the ways programs have, or should, target teenagers.

According to rational choice theory, an individual makes decisions by assessing the relative value of the options available to her. She weighs the costs of behavior against the benefits. A young woman must have access to accurate information in order to make an effective, informed choice among various options. Is knowledge truly power? Will it lead to behavior change? Are there situations in which a young adult with a reasonable knowledge base will still engage in risky behavior? Surveys of AIDS and contraceptive knowledge show that most young adults understand the basic concepts and issues associated with sexually transmitted diseases and other outcomes related to unprotected sexual activity; however, many still engage in risky behaviors.

In the 1989 Secondary School Student Health Risk Survey (SSSHRS), a survey of 8,098 high school–aged teenagers, 98 percent of them identified three of the highest risk activities associated with contracting HIV.[2] In general, teenagers display more knowledge of the means of HIV transmission and risk groups than the medical and health facts about AIDS. Furthermore, they want more medical information from physicians and prefer talking with either medical professionals or friends rather than with their parents.[3] Studies such as these clearly indicate that most teenagers, from different racial-ethnic groups, socioeconomic backgrounds, and regions of the country, have some basic knowledge of AIDS and HIV.

Beth Richie (1990) argues that black women of all ages are overrepresented among people with AIDS because of a lack of prevention programs, inadequate primary health care, and an absence of adequate support, both social and emotional.[4] She criticizes the lack of institutional supports that increase lasting behavior change and risk reduction. Officials with the National Institutes of Health also recognize that institutional support is important.[5] Underfunded prevention and intervention programs cannot meet the needs of community members. Such programs are often understaffed and overworked; employees have to meet case management as well as administrative needs. Furthermore, inadequate primary health care limits a woman's access to and contact with the health care system as a whole. If she has contracted an STD, is pregnant, or merely needs a check-up, she risks sporadic care. As a result, health problems go undetected and may become life-threatening.

"Cultural" barriers to care also exist. A provider who is not versed in the unique needs of her patients may say or do things that alienate members of the community. Some providers who work with populations of color and/or with poor clients retain stereotypical perceptions of these men and women. They make assumptions about medical questions.[6] These barriers to health promotion initiatives increase the risk faced by low-income black women and Latinas. This point is supported by another research team whose study indicates that adolescents using family planning clinics reported a higher rate of contraceptive use than those who had no preventive health care.[7]

Decisions regarding sexual activity, reproduction, and pregnancy are affected by a range of structural, environmental, and psychosocial mechanisms. How a woman defines her personal risk of HIV infection is influenced by her perceived life options as well as the importance placed on her personal relationships. Feeling in control of her future, developing trust in her partner, and identifying potential choices in her future outside of pregnancy increase the likelihood that a young woman will actively reduce risk. Accurate information, social support, and counseling are necessary for behavior change. Access to preventive medical care by itself is insufficient.

A young woman who does not believe that having unprotected sex and eschewing condoms are risking her current and future life options is less likely to entertain behavior change. Even those who want to alter their behavior will not do so if they are lacking the social or material support necessary to facilitate their changes. AIDS education must therefore provide teenagers with two sets of skills: the tools necessary for acquiring information and the tools that will enable them to change their behavior.

Young black women's racial identities, as well as racism, can influence their sexual identity. Women's sense of racial being is a constant, yet unarticulated, part of their individual identity. Racism further reminds black women of their status. Whether middle-class, working-class, or poor, racism is a presence in their lives. Social class, while not necessarily linked to race and sexuality, certainly modifies the lives of young black women. Experiencing social isolation and alienation, needing control over one's life, mistrusting men, and defining one's future as limited are all outcomes of living with a series of institutional and structural constraints. All of these factors affect how a woman defines and responds to her potential risk. They determine whether she will introduce condoms into a relationship or whether she will define contraceptives as self-protection. Pregnancy and AIDS prevention address these issues. Subtle and more explicit pressures to become pregnant are effective barriers to contraception. The cultural and symbolic meanings of the reproductive and childbearing process must be understood and reflected in AIDS prevention.

Intervention and prevention programs have been varyingly successful in their efforts with teenagers. They have been effective at educating teens about pregnancy and HIV but not at permanently changing behavior. This result is due to the way some initiatives are structured. They disseminate information without addressing or improving environmental factors and opportunity structures that interfere with young women's ability and willingness to change behavior and reduce risk. Additionally, proponents of educational efforts have also confronted resistance and controversy within city departments of health, school systems, and religious institutions, and have faced the scrutiny of parents. Some of the issues faced by teenagers, educators, and outreach workers in New Haven reflect those faced throughout the nation.

Teenagers in New Haven, despite resistance from some parents and interest groups, have a number of resources that provide reproductive, sexual, and AIDS-related information. There is variation regarding the specificity, frequency, and accessibility to information. Many resources are not monitored or evaluated, which explains some of the variation. In some cases, program development is dependent on one person. Schools allow teachers to tailor educational materials more than parents realize. Teenagers are sometimes denied more current or comprehensive information because of their young age. Organizational and infrastructural implications fall outside the scope of this chapter, but it has become apparent that program directors can, and want to, benefit from sharing resources.

Many communities are committed to the implementation of innovative programs for teenagers. Various agencies and community organizations have coordinated efforts over the past fifteen years. Occasionally there is some overlap in effort, but sharing resources is rare because of interorganizational competition and antagonism. Different factions of parents are in opposition over the purpose and content of school initiatives as well as the introduction of programs for teen parents. Religious organizations, as has been reported in many cities,[8] have been slow to tackle the AIDS issue from pulpits out of fear of sending a non-Christian message to youth.

Teenage girls know about the means of HIV transmission and infection and about the importance of using only condoms for protection. They report being inundated by information ranging from the classroom to public service announcements and media coverage of national stories. Being overwhelmed has had an unintended result: desensitization. Conversations with young women illustrated that information eventually reaches the point of diminishing returns. A kind of backlash results. In the end, they want to avoid thinking about AIDS. AIDS seems to constrain and overwhelm their lives. In response to this, they ignore and deny their personal risks in the hopes that AIDS will disappear. The backlash takes the form of not using condoms and engaging in behaviors that increase the risk of infection.

What young women know about AIDS is different from how they feel about AIDS. Although many know of the means of transmission and protection, their choice to identify their risk and protect themselves was tempered by what AIDS symbolized. Just as pregnancy, motherhood, virginity, and sexuality have conventional social value and meaning, so do HIV and AIDS. What AIDS symbolizes for them often transforms how they defined their own risk of contracting HIV. It represents things young adults wish to avoid addressing in their own lives.

Young adults are usually viewed as a unique group requiring special educational strategies. Strategies used to encourage avoiding teenage pregnancy have been extended to include AIDS prevention.[9] Clinics and other organizations distribute condoms and encourage their consistent usage. Other projects emphasize expanding knowledge and influencing attitudes using much of the same curriculum as in traditional sex education classes.

The segment of the adolescent population missed by these initiatives includes homeless teenagers, high school dropouts, and teenagers who face barriers to commonly available resources. Outreach programs are only as effective as the individuals who create them and the institutional structures supporting them. Without consistently available resources, many young adults are unable to gain the knowledge necessary for a reduction in risk behavior, nor can they access the services that facilitate these changes.[10]

Sources of AIDS Information: What New Haven Can Teach Us

Discussion over the appropriate role of sex education includes a new array of issues since the advent of AIDS.[11] From conversations with parents, teachers, and students, it became apparent that this debate touches upon sensitive, difficult topics. These comments, from teachers and young women, reflect how difficult the issue has become.

> Parents do not want to know about any sex ed in their children's classrooms. They fear that their kids will be taken over by the spirit and start having sex in the hallways and then start missing class as a result. I'm being a little flip about this, but it's true in a lot of cases.

I think we have no business introducing sex in school. We have taken on a parenting role, and that can be dangerous. I would not want a stranger telling my son or daughters about sex and other personal things.

I'm happy we do sex classes. I learned about AIDS and things. I liked it when some outsider people came in. Many friends don't know the first thing about anything, and they could use more information.

That gets me embarrassed. In the seventh grade, when we had to talk about the birds and the bees, [it] made me feel weird. I don't like talking in class about that. I don't even talk that way to my friends!

Some teachers and parents disregard the possibility that their children and/or their children's peers are already sexually active and thus in immediate need of comprehensive information. This level of denial can shape the content of curricula prepared for the classroom. For example,

While AIDS education has been mandated in several states, many of the educational efforts provide only biomedical information and use fear as a means of trying to control adolescents' sexual behaviors. . . . Many program efforts have also skirted sexuality issues. In a review of 18 published school AIDS curricula, the CDC found that two-thirds advocated a one-class/one-hour session; one quarter did not address condom use; and only 22% of the curricula emphasized that it is behavior which places individuals at risk for HIV.[12]

Even parents who acknowledge that their teenagers may be sexually active can express resistance to a sex ed curriculum that covers more than physiological change. Questions concerning the level of detail necessary for sex ed classes have been raised by teenagers, too. The boundaries between information to be shared in the public (school) and private (family) spheres are less tangible.[13] What constitutes excessive information for adolescents? Who is responsible for making this decision and enforcing the boundaries?

This debate reflects the assumption that both the source and the explicitness of sexual information directly influences whether a teenager will engage in sexual activity.[14] A common objection to introducing sex education to teenagers is that it implicitly permits them to become sexually active. Under the specter of AIDS, this objection gains urgency. Recently, a nationally known sex educator won a lawsuit filed by a group of Boston area high school students and their parents who claimed that her explicit message constituted sexual harassment.[15] Public exchanges over sexuality might be interpreted as a societal sanctioning of promiscuity: Allowing these exchanges with the added threat of HIV infection is too risky for some individuals. Thus, the stakes associated with sex education have increased.

These increased stakes extend to determining who should provide sex education. Traditionally, sex education has referred to curricula taught in junior high or high school classrooms.[16] Obviously, a young woman can learn about sex and contraception through other avenues. Friends, peers, relatives, music, television, and magazines are all potential sources for information. These various sources can shape, whether actively or not, a young woman's outlook concerning her sexuality; there are many situations outside the realm of sex education where young women learn about sexuality and reproduction.

When asked to outline where they learn about AIDS, HIV, and sex, the majority of young women in the sample were surprisingly nonspecific. They stated that they assumed it was from school or from friends. Susie, a seventeen-year-old high school senior, explained that "you just know about AIDS because it's everywhere . . . on TV, in the news. . . . [You] can't avoid hearing about it. That way everyone knows at least the basics." For Allison, the sources were also unclear. "One day AIDS was just there. I'm not sure where I first heard about it. Probably in school, I guess. But also from some of my girlfriends. We're all up on that stuff, like how you get it and how to tell who has it.[17] Also television, too."

Few of these young women actually reported a specific person or group of persons who explicitly discussed AIDS with them. Although they claim to have received some form of AIDS information, in the majority of cases this instruction constituted being told that AIDS should be avoided and that it is "bad to have." In keeping with surveys of AIDS and contraceptive knowledge, it has been easier to determine what these young women know rather than what their source(s) of information are.[18]

This question of the source(s) and content of information is especially important if effective projects are to be developed that inform youth and prepare them to make decisions in potentially compromising circumstances. It is also important because outreach workers and health care providers can be even more effective when they are aware of the various ways youth learn about AIDS and how influential these sources are. My assumption is that informal information networks may have a lasting influence on young women because they are incorporated into the daily experience of these individuals. These networks are so integrated that most teenagers could not identify specific sources of AIDS information. Casual conversations as well as observing others' behavior can influence what a young woman may do in the future.

The young women were uniformly critical of the formal, institution-alized sources of AIDS-related information and suggested a number of ways to increase their effectiveness. Ninety percent strongly believed that schools should provide intensive, explicit sex education classes. What appealed to them most was the prospect of having peer counsel-ors and educators to talk to.[19] Also, most wished that they were able to talk to their parents about these issues.

What remains unclear, however, is whether teenagers would will-ingly approach their parents even if they were willing to discuss such issues with their children. In previous chapters, I described how un-comfortable teenagers were with the prospect of discussing personal reproductive matters with any adult, especially a parent. Their discom-fort was reinforced by their parents, who also avoided specific conver-sations out of fear that they would have to discuss their own pasts or that their interest would be construed as endorsing sexual activity. Those who discussed sex-related things with their parents were also more likely to feel comfortable with their sexuality. This attitude made them more proactive in obtaining information from trustworthy and confidential sources. Conversations, though, were rarely initiated by the teenagers. Young women were able to ask questions and include their parents in their information-gathering process once their parents expressed interest or concern in them.

Considering the scope of sources available to the "typical" young woman within her social environment, the task of determining the rel-ative influence of each source is at best difficult. A more realistic ana-lytic approach involves (1) focusing on how young women respond to the information they have received from these sources and (2) discuss-ing which sources they credit with being most influential in their own lives and personal decisions.

Parents and Families

Whether intentionally or not, parents and other relatives influence a young woman's emerging sexual identity. Part of this process involves internalizing the images and values present in her home environment. Parental attitudes, beliefs, and behavior provide young women with a framework in which they negotiate their lives. A notable exception is AIDS education. Few of the young women reported learning about AIDS from their parents, particularly their fathers. In fact, most re-ported the topic was never addressed beyond being told to "not get it."

At the same time however, a few feel comfortable talking with their parents about other reproductive and sexual issues. These discussions often assumed the form of conversations about boyfriends or the importance of contraception. If these young women and their parents were so comfortable, why did they still avoid discussions about HIV and AIDS?

As Rhonda explained, "My mother knows I'm taking the pill, but we don't need to talk any more about it than that. Anyways, she'd be bugging if AIDS ever came up. . . . What would I be doing to get the HIV virus and stuff?" She alluded to a carefully preserved blanket of denial concerning her mother's assessment of Rhonda's risk: "So, like how do we talk about it, you know. She doesn't like me having sex, but at least I'm trying to avoid a baby. There is no need to go worrying about AIDS. That's what she'd say, I think."

Though this comment is not an indictment of parents, Rhonda's description does reflect a continuing resistance among some parents to recognizing that more teenagers are engaging in very high-risk behavior and are doing so willingly. Other teenagers described infrequent attempts to discuss AIDS-related issues. For example, one common strategy involved asking them what they had learned in school. "My father asked me about the visit from the clinic lady," explained one participant. "He really got me, because he never asks me anything, except when I go out with a guy, then he's all over *him*! So he wanted to know about whether this lady talked about weird things and if we learned about condoms. When I tell him yes about the condoms, he kind of smiles and says, 'Good; boys will try to skip condoms. You don't want AIDS.' That was the whole talk."

In spite of attention to the importance of parental influence or adult role models in teenagers' lives, few initiatives have managed to include parents in the adolescents' educational process.

> Given the importance of the family unit as a support system for the aspirations and accomplishments of children moving through the educational system, and its potential as a source of sexual socialization of children, it follows that the task of reducing the risk of adolescent pregnancy [and the associated risk of contracting an STD] by means of educational programs could be more successfully accomplished by utilizing the support and reinforcement potential that parents have. Sex education programs might therefore seek to forge a new partnership between instructors, mothers and daughters by including mothers in the educational process. . . . Involving parents might also function to diffuse a significant portion of parental resistance to sex and contraception education programs in a given school district . . . and improving the chances for success in obtaining the program objectives.[20]

Although this approach would not be intended to replace the parental role, it may enable parents to broach sensitive issues more comfortably with their children.

One of the most critical psychosocial characteristics found among many teenagers is a need to distinguish themselves from their parents and their parents' values. Given this point it is unrealistic to assume that teenagers are likely to seek out their parents for detailed discussions of either sexuality or STDs. Furthermore, there is little motivation to encourage parents to engage in frank discussion, because their own sexuality is traditionally "off limits" to children. By making parent training available through schools, some of this discomfort might be alleviated, enabling parents to initiate intimate conversation more comfortably with their children.

Friends and Peers

Young women reported discussing AIDS and HIV with their friends, though not necessarily within an educational context. Even in a trusted cohort, they were acutely aware of the need for image management. In fact, "it isn't a good idea to bring this [AIDS] up all the time, in case people start wondering if you have it." Conversations often centered on speculation over who had contracted an STD. Gossip on dating and relationships includes talking about sexual activity, pregnancy, and disease. Whenever AIDS was raised in conversations concerning personal relationships, it was in conjunction with condom use.

What does it mean for these young women to talk with their friends about AIDS and sex? A vast body of research confirms that teenage girls discuss personal issues with each other. Additional data suggest that the influence of peers on behavior has illustrated how important "opinion leaders" can be in public health efforts to change behavior.[21] What form do these conversations take? Raising issues with friends does not mean that a teenager is seeking information or advice from others. As this age period is one of self-discovery and increased independence in preparation for adulthood, references to one's private life may simply be a way to generate emotional support or approval.

Furthermore, there is a difference between regularly sharing information and sporadically talking about sexuality and reproduction. This distinction clearly has to be made when researching the influence peers have on each other. The structure provided by after school programs and other institutionally created peer groups is artificial to a certain extent and cannot reflect the way teenagers' social groups are composed. I did observe that the dynamics of peer groups shaped what a young woman would share and how she communicated with others.

The nature of information participants shared with each other was dependent on who the audience was. The young women were more likely to seek support and advice from their closest friends. In rare situations did they express a willingness to delve into their most personal thoughts, concerns, and questions. When asked about her relationship with her closest friend, one eighteen-year-old said, "I know that Regina is down with me, and she got my back. We talk and shit, and we share things." This relationship did not include intimate discussions of sexuality, particularly AIDS-related topics. "Nah, talking like that would be nasty. We all know who's a freak and who's disease. Most I'd say is about my man dogging me with another woman one time. . . . But not much 'cause you got to watch for the hoochies."

The social isolation and alienation experienced by the poor and working poor teenagers may have some effect on their protectiveness. Even with closest friends there is the chance of betrayal over a man or emotional abandonment. Appearing to be strong and independent thus extends into their most intimate female relationships and alters their willingness to seek out advice.

Friends do share information and communicate expectations since beliefs are manifested in behavior. For example, young adolescent mothers often expressed that their curiosity over pregnancy was piqued by close friends' or relatives' own reproductive experiences. Role models can subtly influence both the knowledge a young woman obtains and how she acts on the information. For Rochelle, her girlfriend's sister was her role model and mentor. This woman, who was twenty-one, was called on for advice:

> So, like Lavonne is my girl but Felicia's got more sense. She's Lavonne's older sister and she's been there. I can talk about whatever I want and I do. . . . We don't get all into that [AIDS], but she tells me about some of her friends who got sick and how messed up they got. She told me upfront that AIDS will get you if you don't use jimmys and that dying that way is worse than anything she ever saw.

Felicia had recently seen a former boyfriend who had AIDS and was very ill. Rochelle believed that Felicia's talk, which was atypical, was inspired by what she had seen. Felicia's graphic description of the physical effects of AIDS disturbed Rochelle and, in her words, "makes me want to be careful more." Whether this awareness will last remains to be seen.

The Popular Media

In New Haven, young adults also have access to formal and informal sources for information about AIDS and sexuality. The methods used to communicate with youth range from the mainstream to the unusual. Public service announcements (PSAs) are broadcast on television and radio. Often the text is tailored to target a specific segment of the audience. Two radio stations that play dance music and rhythm and blues have used well-known personalities to educate the public about a variety of issues, from teen pregnancy and responsible parenthood to the association between unprotected sexual activity and/or intravenous drug use and HIV.

Popular magazines—for example, *YSB* (*Young Sisters and Brothers*), *Essence*, and *Vibe*—occasionally provide a forum for discussion among black teenagers. Though each of these targets a unique readership, they all reflect the cultural distinctiveness of blacks. *YSB* and *Vibe* focus on popular culture, and frequently showcase articles written by teenagers' peers and role models. These pieces deal with relationship issues, sexuality, and drug and alcohol use through their emphasis on adolescent self-expression.

Essence, though more aggressively geared toward college-educated, middle-class black women, is also popular among teenage girls. Because of the age of its intended readership, this magazine tends to deal with sexuality more explicitly than the other two periodicals. Because articles on AIDS and sex-related articles are regularly published, the fact that they are read by a sizable group of teenagers illustrates their potential as an alternate resource for these young women.

Occasionally, teenagers referred to magazine features addressing sexual issues. What appeared to appeal most to them were television programs. Music videos, though blamed for communicating overtly sexual images for young adults, were rarely credited with teaching youth about their sexuality. They viewed television images as pure entertainment. In fact, some initiated discussions about the negative way they thought women were represented. I found no instances where what they saw in a video was directly translated into their personal lives. In fact, they are so accustomed to highly sexual images, and to PSAs that they have become desensitized to these messages. They are more interested in seeing which personalities are used in the most current media campaigns than in the content.

Clinics and Health Care Agencies

The City Department of Health and community agencies are involved in outreach efforts in many neighborhoods throughout New Haven. Various health clinics and hospitals actively engage in education and outreach. Outreach workers literally engage people in conversation on street corners and organize formal presentations by invitation. Clinics distribute pamphlets in waiting rooms and sponsor activities geared toward "AIDS awareness" (e.g., World AIDS Day events).

Two of the agencies specifically targeting youth at risk and providing after-school activities are also dedicated to disseminating AIDS-related information to young adults and teenagers. Coordinators for these programs have incorporated statistics on sexual activity, contraceptive use, and STD rates in their curricula. One technique used with teenagers is the distribution of comic books. These bilingual (Spanish and English) comics offer commentaries on the problems and questions many teenagers have concerning HIV and AIDS. In one story line, a young man is forced to confront his own homophobia when he discovers that his brother is both HIV positive and gay. In addition, agencies use videotapes, guest speakers, field trips, and games to make the information more relevant to clients.

Agency officials shared with me anecdotal evidence of behavior change in their clients. Teen girls who opted to avoid future pregnancies, who talked to partners about condoms, and who sought regular gynecological care were three popular examples of success stories. Teenagers who voluntarily participated in these programs were more motivated to incorporate new knowledge into their lives. The others, considered at risk for health and other problems, resisted counselors' efforts.

Schools

The Board of Education has mandated that all New Haven middle and high schools should provide one term of sex education for students.[22] When asked about this, both students and educators expressed frustration over the inadequacy of the curriculum. Frustration seems to be a common thread connecting educators throughout the nation. One high school teacher described an incident in a colleague's classroom:

> Some speakers from [an AIDS education program staffed and run by medical school students] was invited by _____ to speak in his class. They were to talk about what AIDS and HIV were and why sex has become so complicated in the '90s. When they were brought to the classroom, he locked the door and told them that they could not discuss anything involving sex or deviant acts because it might influence the kids. I suppose his concern was that they may start engaging in all sorts of behaviors. Can you believe that he really thought that they were not sexually active already? Just another case of denial, like many parents. That's

why we can't get regular sex ed in any of the schools, despite what people
will tell you.

Students reported that schools were unreliable sources of information.
As in the above example, much of the curriculum could be tailored by
the teachers with no repercussions from school administrators. In
other cases, students claim that in a given term they were exposed to
fewer than five classes focused on sex and contraception. What is ironic
is that school-based clinics were often viewed as the only reliable
sources for information for high school students. As of 1990 there were
178 school-based clinics nationwide in junior and senior high schools.[23]
In most cases the clients are low-income minorities who use them for
primary health care needs.

The ongoing controversy over the role of sex education in the classroom has continued. This debate includes concern over the distribution
of condoms in a few local high schools and the recent institution of a
child care center at one high school for teen mothers who are still in
school. Parents have been quoted as criticizing the advent of AIDS education in the schools because it may encourage previously uninterested
youth to engage in sexual activity. AIDS has been introduced into the
sex education debate as an example of attempts to introduce adult issues to a too-young audience. Because AIDS is still frequently associated with homosexuality and drug use, some parents have expressed
concern over exposing their children to these "deviant" groups.

Health educators and teachers in New Haven shared personal stories
of change, but they also expressed frustration over being restricted
from greater involvement with their students. They were frustrated by
parents resisting teacher involvement in such a personal issue; parental
denial of the sexuality of youth causes more problems than solutions.
Comprehensive education cannot lead to change, then, without the co-
operation of parents, educators, outreach workers, city agencies, grass-
roots organizations, and the young men and woman who are targeted.
In the absence of any one of these elements, teenagers are placed at
greater risk of HIV infection.

AIDS educators express interest in more broad-based health care initiatives in the school system. Partly in response to the high rates of
teenage pregnancy and sexually transmitted diseases, these programs
are tailored specifically to some of the needs of the adolescent population. Local high schools offer a variety of initiatives that are affiliated
with their clinics that address issues of sexuality. One clinic cosponsors
a project directed toward young women, especially those of color. It
provides a forum in which participants can talk about any health related issues, particularly ones concerning sexual activity and preg-

nancy. Information is provided, as well as more individualized counseling. The participants constitute a support network.

Imagining AIDS and HIV: Social and Clinical Knowledge

What one knows about HIV and AIDS and what one feels and believes about them are different issues. People have images of what AIDS can do to the body and how emotionally challenging living with AIDS might be. Sympathy and empathy for persons living with AIDS may not evolve into personal commitments to behavior change and risk reduction. In chapter 1 I summarized the way the social meaning of AIDS transformed during the 1980s. This transformation resulted in redefining risk groups and risk behaviors and in identifying HIV as a national crisis.

Social valuation of disease and health occurs among young men and women as well. AIDS has been assigned distinctive medical and social meanings. It is primarily defined as a disease that victimizes others. Teenagers have been inundated with information concerning the deadly nature of HIV and AIDS. Being overwhelmed with information through public forums has desensitized young women to AIDS. They depersonalize the disease by limiting the potential threat it poses in their lives.

Addressing HIV Infection: What AIDS Symbolizes

Perspectives on HIV are shaped by a girl's assessment of her own risk level and by the "ranking" of her risk in comparison with other factors in her life. Naturally her response to issues of life and death will depend on whether she sees herself as essentially mortal or immortal. But even if she can respond to the message that HIV is deadly and to be avoided and even if she knows she has been at risk, a young woman may still minimize the need for protection because she cannot reconcile the reality of her situation with her idealized view of what her situation ought to be.

What does HIV mean, and how do young women connect HIV and AIDS to their own lives? During a week-long debate with some girls, I asked them to describe what HIV was. I was interested to see how they identified the virus and/or AIDS as a disease: whether they saw HIV and AIDS as something that happens to other people, as a dangerous presence in their communities, or as a more personal issue. At issue is whether they have internalized the information concerning AIDS in a way that would at least facilitate accurate and appropriate concern for their personal risk.

In each case I began a conversation with a basic question: "What is HIV, and what is AIDS?" This query prompted many different kinds of responses.

> AIDS is a disease you can get from sex, or dirty needles. Anyone can get it these days, so you have to be kinda careful with yourself, you know. I think HIV is like the first step in AIDS.

> AIDS can kill you, HIV can't.

> So HIV virus is a sort of sickness you catch in having sex with unclean people. Other things can get you HIV, like too much drugs or being around too many of those kinds . . . Homosexuals and stuff bring HIV the most.

> I don't know specifically, just that as long as I stay with my boyfriend and don't do any drugs, like crank or herb, I'll be safe.

These descriptions, apart from their range in accuracy, all deal in medical terms. All those who described HIV or AIDS did so in terms of infection, disease, and sickness. Many identified AIDS as "the end of a road" or as "a death sentence." The visual impact of the "silence = death" campaign on teenagers has been critical in their defining AIDS as deadly. Public service announcements and other media treatments of HIV and AIDS have effectively brought this message home as well. The irony is that defining HIV as potentially causing death has reshaped how teenagers determine whether they need to change behavior.

Young women do worry about AIDS, even in terms of personal risk. They do so, however, in ways that highlight why knowledge is not resulting in different "lifestyles." AIDS education has shown young women that AIDS is a social problem because it is an incurable disease, it can be communicated through a range of legal and illegal "leisure time" or private activities, and virtually anyone could be exposed to some level of risk. They have also learned that HIV and AIDS can be avoided through abstinence, monogamy, condom use, and refusal to use illegal drugs.

Even with all of this information available to them, what is missing is a critical link to their personal worlds. Resistance to personalizing the possibility of AIDS infection was a common problem among women.

I don't know what AIDS would mean to me. I don't think I'll get it, even though it's around.

What are my chances of being infected? You mean now? None. I am always careful. . . . Condoms are there for a reason.

I just can't get into that.

As long as I know who I am with, and he knows about me, I'll have no problems; anyone can get it, I suppose. Even me. But that hasn't happened and it won't.

Although they have learned that HIV infection can essentially be avoided, they tend to minimize the threat of personal risk and thus ignore taking self-protective measures.

Control becomes transposed into denial and inaction. Asserting control is defined as picking "AIDS-free" partners, probably one of the riskiest options available to a sexually active person. As long as girls believe that such a shift in behavior can reduce their risk substantially, they will have little motivation to alter basic attitudes and beliefs (which is the only route to long-term behavior change).

Obviously young women have internalized the message concerning AIDS and are responding by making personal changes. While risk avoiders define AIDS in ways that echo those women who do not use condoms or reduce other risks, they are apparently defining personal risk in different ways. Those who lower risk are more likely to see AIDS as an eventual death sentence. Infection is connected with finality and a loss of opportunities.

The thought of getting AIDS scares me. Does it hurt? How long can you live with it? I don't like thinking in those terms because it depresses me. I am basically terrified.

I don't know anyone with AIDS, but I've heard about it. You look fine, at first, then everything starts to go. Imaging one night of fun in exchange for a lifetime of torment. Actually, it isn't even a whole lifetime.

Fear of infection and understanding of the finality of the disease still do not guarantee risk reduction. Other factors must be involved. Most important is the perception and recognition of risk; to what extent do teenagers perceive AIDS as a personal risk?

Reassessing and Redefining Risk

One of the central contentions in this book has been that definitions of risky behavior are relative. Health organizations such as the Centers for Disease Control have documented the kinds of risky activities associated with contracting or communicating HIV.[24] In determining what constitutes risky sexual behavior, these agencies use evaluative categories that reflect one particular social reality. This reality (limiting sexual partners, using condoms, avoiding drugs, and abstinence) may or may not resonate with young adults. The social environments in which teenagers live influence their attitudes, beliefs, and actions. A teenager with a value system similar to the one promoted by health care providers and outreach workers would likely respond to interventions and educational initiatives.

The social reality of poor and working poor teenagers can negate, or cancel out, their commitment to behavior change. Being surrounded by images of poverty, young parents, and drug use may enhance feelings of despair and hopelessness. Since risk is defined in relation to the totality of a teenager's social existence, not having strong resources to counteract the negative aspects of this reality can result in her not minimizing her personal risk.

> Interventions will count for little in the absence of realistic opportunities for disadvantaged young people to become participating members of society. . . . [B]oth the psychological and social conditions of their lives, and the economic realities, must be altered.[25]

The combination of information, social support, and counseling is essential for lasting change.[26]

In encouraging risk reduction, effective educational and outreach programs should account for the social relevance of public health norms to the community being targeted.[27] Attention to the sociocultural contexts of reproductive choice and the definitions of relative risk have been cited as contributing to the success of interventions.[28] The compensation for changes in behavior needs to be relevant to a young woman's own social situation. This also means that both the AIDS-related messages and the strategies for change would reflect her cultural and socioeconomic background.[29] Whatever culturally based messages will effectively communicate the importance of attitude and behavior change would be more appealing to a black teenager. Thus, the tools and skills necessary for initiating and maintaining changes extend beyond an individual's personal strengths and abilities.[30] Factors including the cultural meaning of womanhood and the related importance of conception, childbearing, the need for intimacy through sexual contact and one's assessment of future options ultimately affect whether a woman can, and will, confront her own risk of infection.

Risk is primarily defined in relation to access to opportunity, perceived life option, and a young woman's need for an intimate or sexual relationship. Determining what constitutes risky behavior also means identifying the complicated array of risks and challenges (both emotional and institutional) young women experience that are not directly correlated with contracting HIV. For example, in spite of her knowledge, if a teenager sees herself as invulnerable, she will not be inclined to reduce the potential risk of exposure she faces. Teenagers who witnessed death and physical violence in their communities were forced to face the reality of their own mortality.

> Folks get messed with all the time. You hear about this one being beaten up or that one getting into a fight. I just try to stay out of folks' way to protect myself. Even that doesn't always work. Sometime ago, this girl starts telling people that she wants to get me, take me down, and I don't know why. Now I have to protect myself. I know what can happen if you don't.

Teenagers normally responded by claiming that they would challenge this norm by either surviving the most unbeatable odds or expecting death. A young woman who has become this cynical[31] may also ignore what she knows about HIV/AIDS because she has become desensitized to risk: "Given an existence where problems such as citizenship status, poverty or lack of health resources are prevalent, a person may develop a fatalistic attitude of 'if one thing doesn't get me, another will' so that AIDS prevention seems unimportant."[32]

I have been arguing that there is not only a schism between adults' and teenagers' definitions of risk but also distinctions among the young women themselves. When women's view of risk varies from pregnancy to HIV infection to nothing and when their life histories can include anything from physical and emotional violence to functional and emotionally intact families, it becomes obvious that no one program can be all-serving. The challenge then becomes presenting information in a way that appeals to the widest variety of backgrounds and perspectives without sacrificing the ultimate goal: changing behavior.[33]

Instilling a sense of responsibility for one's well-being is an important strategy used by successful programs.[34] Enabling young women to define their own worldviews, particularly the role of sex and sexuality, allows them room to define what risk means to them. Some teenage women value sex for creating intimate relationships, whereas others see it in clear power terms. Asking, not telling a young woman, about her sexuality places her in the position of actor. In contrast, telling her to change without determining whether she wants to is a tactic destined to fail. This is relevant to defining what risk is because at some basic level "risk" refers to something negative, something unacceptable. For a teenager to absorb her new knowledge and subsequently alter her behavior, she has to agree that the targeted behavior is negative and unhealthy.

Where, then, does the risk lie for most young women—in the behavior itself or in the outcomes associated with the behavior? Furthermore, what outcomes will be of immediate concern to a young adult? A young woman's generalized definition of risk often differs from her assessment of her personal risk status. Laurine knew what she called the "do's and don'ts of AIDS": "You don't have sex with someone, or something, you don't know. Stay away from drugs, or at least be careful about it. You do talk about it and use a condom. Don't have sex drunk. Don't share needles. Do have an AIDS test if you've had a lot of sex. Don't think you can't get it, because anyone can." At the same time, she admitted to drinking at parties and having sex with different men: "I know enough to know when I've gone too far. I only sleep with guys I know, and I know about their backgrounds, so I am not in any real danger." Her logic has given her a false sense of security; consequently, she rarely uses condoms.

Factors influencing whether one will engage in or avoid high-risk activities can be individual or interpersonal ones.[35] For example, there is the issue of others' perceptions of one's risk. A young woman's assessment of the importance of these behavioral changes will be negatively affected. She may be more worried about how others will label her if she insists on using a condom or alters her sexual behavior. She may in fact consider others' critical responses to her behavior change as the greater risk instead of identifying multiple sexual partners or drug/alcohol use as risky. Girls who depend on their boyfriend for a sense of identity will be more concerned about keeping him happy than about health and mortality. They fear alienating their partners and being abandoned. These girls have to be taught how to assert themselves with their partners.[36] Both risk and related outcomes can refer to behavior, attitudes, beliefs, and lifestyle, which could mean anything from providing people with information to preventing transmission or changing behavior. What is meant by this approach needs to be clearly identified by both participants and providers.

How Effective Are HIV and AIDS Prevention Programs?

As stipulated by the AIDS Risk Reduction Model, for newly acquired knowledge to be translated into action (protection from HIV infection), an individual needs to believe in her own efficacy (ability to influence events that happen in her environment) as well as a supportive network that facilitates her change. Prevention programs and interventions are rarely equipped to deal with these stages of a young woman's behavioral change. This is true for young women with some social support as well as those lacking it.

Family life courses, available to expectant teenagers and teenage mothers, normally include components addressing these issues.[37] A health center's programs are dedicated to augmenting the participants' life skills; the providers have acknowledged that the basic skills addressed in the curriculum may determine whether the young women successfully negotiate through their adolescence. Improving interpersonal skills, learning how to find employment (particularly in a city with a depressed economy), developing nutrition programs that are sensitive to the financial constraints of clients, and discussing physiological and reproductive processes are all relevant for a teenager's survival. The imperative to translate HIV knowledge and the need for safer sex to verbal and behavioral "repertoires" becomes real when these other issues are concurrently addressed.[38]

The continuing danger lies in community-based resistance to recognizing young adults' sexuality and the range of influences on their choices and actions. The controversy over the merits of school-based prevention initiatives show how much resistance there is to the reality that teens are sexually active and need nonfamilial resources. Barriers and impediments to participation in programs and a lack of receptiveness to outreach have institutional, social, and philosophical (values-based) sources.[39] If members of a community resist recognizing what their youth do or if adults attempt to address only one part of the problem, the majority of teenagers will not have the resources necessary to make life-advancing decisions.[40]

Measuring Risk Reduction and Behavior Change

What benchmarks indicate the success of an intervention? In creating an effective program, Cates (1991) recommends including skill building along with the provision of a knowledge base.[41] Without the skills to both initiate change and resist peer pressure, knowledge will not be translated into safe behaviors (this is, in Cates's terms, "action-oriented" education). According to the National Coalition of Advocates for Students, programs need three elements: comprehensive health or family life courses, attention to the chronological and developmental age of students, and an emphasis on healthy behavior.[42]

Though debate frequently arises over proposed initiatives, fewer data are available on the measurement of program success. In studies measuring the effectiveness interventions, the majority rely on two kinds of indicators. One type involves comparisons of questionnaires measuring AIDS-related knowledge before and after the intervention.[43] A second category compares rates of health outcomes such as pregnancy and HIV infection and/or behavioral outcomes such as contraceptive use in sites targeted by an intervention with control groups.[44] Longitudinal studies concern the length of time behavior change lasts. Usually program participants are followed up between six months to a year after the program ends.

None of these kinds of indicators can sufficiently measure the residual effects of interventions and preventive programs. This would require a long-term follow up of behavior change lasting at least as long as the asymptomatic period following infection: seven to ten years. Most available measurements are of knowledge change and not attitude change.[45] Showing that participants develop positive attitudes about condoms does not mean that they are more likely to believe they should use them.

Does short-term change count in the same manner as long-term change? A number of national and regional studies report that behavior change resulted from prevention initiatives, but if these changes are temporary, the effectiveness of the program must be questioned. Different levels of data thus need to be collected. Short- and long-term changes have to be measured, along with the factors contributing to each type of change.

What constitutes true behavior change in AIDS prevention, and is this ultimately what programs are expected to accomplish? Understanding program goals and expectations provides some framework for identifying and defining positive changes among participants. Unfortunately, in many cases there is "no clearly defined program and sequence of research in the area of sexual behavior and its modification."[46] From my field project, one fact has emerged.

In spite of the conflicting information and evaluation concerns, we cannot dispute that interventions have successfully educated youth about AIDS. There is great variation in what young people know, but they are all aware of HIV and basic risks associated with behavior. These victories can be measured with objective instruments. What is difficult to determine is behavior change. Is a young woman who goes from never using condoms to using them sporadically an example of a success? Her behavior change might be associated with her new knowledge, but she still faces great risk. Should pregnancy and sex ed programs be counted as AIDS interventions? Logically, a young woman who wants to avoid becoming pregnant may still face risk, but does her education make her more receptive to AIDS prevention?

When asked to evaluate their programs, health care workers and social service agencies described individual stories of success. In some cases, young women decided to postpone future pregnancies until they were more established. In other situations, young women tested on AIDS knowledge showed substantial improvement. All of this is exciting and offers hope, but the results are nonscientific. Evidence from the field is important for both the "expert" and the participant, but it has much less meaning for the social scientist who has only second hand knowledge of the young women affected.

New Haven's community agencies, as with most agencies throughout the United States, deal in the present when evaluating their programs. They are mostly concerned with short-term improvement and program recidivism for practical reasons. Most agencies operate in a reactive way, where time is limited. Agencies have little time and few resources to conduct extensive follow-up on former participants. The same is true of clinics and school-based sex education programs. As long as a sizable percentage of participants improve the scope of their knowledge, the program is deemed successful.

In acknowledging the complexity of evaluation, the Government Accounting Office (GAO) has recommended that

> mechanisms be put into place both to evaluate ongoing programs and to test, by using experimental paradigms, the efficacy of theoretically derived behavior change programs. . . . Evaluations of prevention efforts and models are largely descriptive and uncontrolled. The initial urgency of the epidemic required that programs be put into place; perhaps time and energy were not initially sufficient to support controlled evaluations as well.[47]

Planning, implementing, and evaluating programs require time and financial resources that many agencies do not have. Community workers' option is to emphasize implementation because their intent is to encourage change in even one person. Ironically, without having had access to the literature, the programs I encountered incorporated many of the strategies recommended in the literature. Sensitivity to emotional and chronological age of clients, cultural referents, and attention to structural barriers to change have enabled agencies to appeal to their young clients.

Where Do We Go from Here?

Prevention initiatives can be categorized by their content and aims. Some provide basic health information, while others emphasize a change in behavior and/or attitudes. Because this disease is essentially communicated through certain interactive behaviors, the ultimate goal of AIDS education is to change an individual's actions. However, as I have already argued, behavior change requires more than providing information. It is problematic to assume that "risky behavior reflects a lack of knowledge, misinformation or deficiencies in understanding. . . . Educational programs designed to simply disseminate relevant facts about AIDS often fail to change attitudes or prejudices because they neglect consideration of the intense emotional reactions elicited by this syndrome."[48]

Information on sexuality and sexual behavior is often disseminated through interventions and educational programs. Often intervention refers to activity initiated during a crisis, whereas education is defined as a preventive measure. Research on AIDS education has identified several avenues through which information is shared with teenagers; these sources range from classrooms to street corner outreach workers and clinics. In my view, less formal sources of information are also available that are equally important. For example, popular media (television, music, and magazines) and peer groups are highly influential sources of information. Whatever social resources are available to a young woman are likely to strongly influence what she learns and how she assimilates the information.

For information to result in transformative behavior, a young woman needs a reliable source for facts, a social network that supports behavior change, and strong problem-solving skills.[49] Any effort to change behavior must focus on getting people to change their attitudes and teaching them how to maintain those changes. This result is most possible when social norms that dictate or guide the course of daily interactions are supportive of change.[50] Teenagers need educational initiatives that improve their HIV/AIDS prevention skills.[51] They need a knowledge base to deal with prevention-related decisions, and they need skills to resist peer pressure. Then they can effectively translate knowledge into safe behaviors.

As Joyce Ladner (1987) has claimed, the only way to decrease the rates of teenage pregnancy and risk of STDs effectively is by focusing on prevention rather than intervention. Targeting the behaviors associated with becoming pregnant and contracting STDs is a necessary but insufficient requirement for lasting change. For risky behaviors to be reduced on a long-term basis, preventive measures must also address the root problems associated with early sexual activity and related outcomes. Therefore, what is necessary is attention to the institutional forces that increase the young women's risk: "Education and training, jobs, sex/family life education, life skills training, peer counseling, male responsibility counseling with equal emphasis on the needs of males and females" are all needed if permanent change is to be effected.[52]

Interventions cannot be defined in narrow terms that do not include structural and institutional changes. Those that are not developed in a sociocultural context have been labeled "passive education": the underlying presumption is that merely presenting a teenager with basic information will elicit the requisite behavior change.[53] Others are also critical of these kinds of interventions because they aim to force behavior change in a particularly invasive way without accounting for the unique environmental factors that distinguish young women's life experiences.

> The argument that a woman who chooses to conceive or continue a pregnancy in the face of possible HIV infection must be either ignorant or unreasonable, or both, reveals the speaker's point of view. It does not acknowledge the leap from bias to moral imperative, and it demonstrates a lack of sensitivity to the profound cultural and social differences between the world of male professionals and the individual worlds of women, especially women of color in the inner cities.[54]

Because interventions implicitly carry a moral imperative to change actions and beliefs, they have to be tailored to the moral worldview of the participants/clients. Acknowledging the sociocultural distinctions in the way teenagers assimilate information and deal with their individual risk improves the effectiveness of preventive programs.

Findings noted throughout this book make the case for broad-sweeping change. Teenagers can effectively reduce their risk of HIV infection when they are offered rewards and mechanisms for change. Intervention cannot be defined in narrow terms that do not include structural and institutional change. Teenagers' risks extend beyond their sexual activity. Drugs, crime, violence, and high school attrition are as much a part of their lives as socializing with friends, dating, working after school, and learning how to become adults. The ways risk, the future, and intimacy are constrained by the entirety of adolescents' experiences have to be reflected in the most basic prevention program.

Social workers, educators, and social scientists are obviously aware of this fact. They discuss skill building, self-esteem, and role models in their attempt to broaden their approach to teen sexuality. They note the ways men influence their clients' decision making. Unfortunately, in some communities, the damage done by living under a state of siege, or by simply being unsure of what the future holds, has already been done. Undoing this damage requires aggressive action. Young black women need educational and job training. They need to develop mediating skills for use in their personal relationships. They need physical spaces where they feel safe and where there are adults they can trust. Only with such systemic change will behavior change be long-lasting.

Programs that do not specifically deal with sexuality or AIDS are essential for prevention. Prevention requires dealing with root causes in order to circumscribe the possibility that social problems will ever emerge. Because inequality, racism, sexism, and class-related phenomena collectively affect sexual behavior, it seems logical to require their elimination in order to fight HIV infection among black teenagers. In programs specifically devoted to sex and AIDS, youth need to be exposed to very explicit information about the costs and benefits of reproductive and sexual behavior. Motherhood, from the fetus's conception to birth and beyond, must be demystified. Teenagers need to learn how transformative behavior change can really be—that they do have more control over their lives than they realize. Condom manufacturers must be included in this change. They have to specifically target a young market. Doing this risks inciting the anger of parents and family values watchdog organizations throughout the nation, which is why behavior change requires community support and involvement and the admission that sex already occurs among young adults and will probably not be eliminated.

A survey of the literature has verified what is already known. In this second decade of the AIDS epidemic, program evaluation is essential if more effective programs are to be created. Though anecdotal evidence and the testimony of participants is not to be ignored, other means of testing the short-, mid-, and long-range effects of initiatives must be devised. Because of the nature of the ways HIV can be communicated, it is advisable that new ways of measurement be devised. Furthermore, educators and outreach workers should consider whether initiatives used for sex education and/or teaching teenagers about other sexually transmitted diseases can or should be used to teach teens about HIV and AIDS. Possibly different social and emotional issues are relevant to AIDS education because the disease cannot be cured.

We thus return to the initial question: What works, in the eyes of the young adults throughout the city? Most support class-based education in addition to other community efforts. This resource alone is not sufficient, however. As some admitted, they are "overeducated" regarding AIDS; teenagers have reached a saturation point from the amount of information they are exposed to. What is important is learning how to use AIDS knowledge in their personal lives; skill building, increased self-control, and peer support cannot evolve from most sex education curricula.

The young women I met were almost unanimous in expressing a need for more peer counselors and educators. Only others in their cohort can understand the challenges and successes faced by contemporary teenagers. Having respected role models in their lives is important to them. They wish for more open relationships with parents and for acceptance of their sexuality. In short, they want to be treated as if they are young adults with individualized beliefs and expectations. When information is provided with respect, not fear or judgment, youth are more responsive and more likely to consider behavior modification. Ultimately, if a young woman believes she has a future ahead of her and if she knows she has support, then she will fight even harder to survive.

8

Just Say No? Reflections on the Reality of AIDS

Will a study of AIDS knowledge, behavior, race, and socioeconomics become obsolete if and when a cure is found? I believe it will still be relevant. It is ironic to note that a still-deadly disease is allowing us the opportunity to confront long-lived social ills. This project demonstrates starkly that the socioeconomic and psychosocial factors associated with risky behaviors are the same factors associated with a wide range of potentially destructive behaviors (including substance abuse and violent crime) and feelings of alienation and isolation.[1] Inequality and community decline can increase feelings of despair and loss of hope, particularly among young adults growing up in communities facing extreme forms of social and fiscal disintegration.[2] I propose that rates of HIV and AIDS infection are associated with certain risky behaviors for a simple reason. Teenagers without a strong sense of community affiliation, who more than other teenagers fear intimate and monogamous relationships and doubt they have a future, are more likely to risk HIV infection.

Immorality and nontraditional values are not persuasive explanations for the trends in infection. Once we argue that risk is associated with behavior, and once the trends in infection cross social categories, a more sophisticated explanation becomes necessary. Although individuals of all ages, races, and socioeconomic backgrounds have tested HIV positive, why is the epidemic so prevalent among people of color? Why are young black and Latino adults contracting HIV and dying from AIDS in such large proportions?

Some might argue that black and Latino teenagers and young adults simply do not like to use condoms or that their levels of sexual activity increase the risk of infection. Though these points may be true to some extent, they do not focus on the fundamental elements behind risk behaviors. As I have emphasized throughout this book, social structure, interpersonal relations, and individual attitudes and beliefs influence the likelihood that a teenager is exposed to HIV, as is true of most risky behaviors. Young adults have faced "perverse demographic trends, deteriorating economies and functional transformations in the structures of urban areas during the past two decades."[3] These urban problems become manifest in the challenges teenagers face, including unemployment, early parenthood, school failure, crime, and substance abuse.

It is no coincidence that the factors associated with early sexual activity and teenage pregnancy are also associated with condom use and risk of exposure to a sexually transmitted disease. Young women of color who are from low-income or poor households face the greatest risk. What is it about their existence that might explain this? Of course, not all poor young women engage in risky behavior, but a disproportionately high number of them do.

Life in poverty, and the way that social reality is represented in the poor's attitudes and behaviors, has been the focus of many sociological and popular culture studies.[4] I, too, am concerned with how social inequality and community decline influence behavior among social groups. Kwame Ture and Charles V. Hamilton (1992) provided a powerful description of the crisis situation they observed in poor black communities in 1967:

> The young drop-out or even high school graduate with an inadequate education, burdened also by the emotional deprivations which are the consequences of poverty, is now on the streets looking for a job. . . . [T]hese are the conditions which create dynamite in the ghettos. And when there are explosions—explosions of frustration, despair and hopelessness—the larger society becomes indignant.[5]

Twenty-five years have passed since the publication of *Black Power*, but the plight of the poor, the existence of those Ture and Hamilton call "colonized people," has remained virtually unchanged. Although this study is not primarily grounded in political economy, I argue that social scientists need to be aware of how the connection between structural factors and poverty can result in outcomes that have been labeled "pathological," "self-destructive," and "epidemic" by conservative theorists and commentators.

How does this discussion relate to AIDS? Young women facing poor life prospects and experiencing loss and isolation force us to recognize the dynamite that is about to explode. Rodrick and Deborah Wallace (1991) describe the living and working conditions of black and Latino poor as preindustrial.[6] Environment is associated with a variety of so-cial-psychological issues that, in turn, influence health behavior and risk taking. A larger social problem rests beneath the surface of reports of high rates of STD infection. There are various ways to resolve feeling a lack of control over one's life, anticipating early death, and needing to be "grown up." How can one gain control over her life in the face of continuing unemployment, poor schools, and high homicide rates among young men between eighteen and twenty-five?[7]

Sexual intercourse and early motherhood cannot be constrained by teachers, parents, employers, police, or any of the many individuals identified as authority figures. Teenagers who do not believe that they can ever achieve success as adults will still look for ways to be per-ceived as such:

> A developmentally poor start, in turn, frequently prepares the ground for early motherhood by encumbering girls with the kinds of psychological boundaries that, within the context of disadvantage, lead to self-limiting choices and self-defeating behavior during the adolescent years. . . . Those who come of age in poverty are given very little margin for error in nego-tiating the tasks of adulthood.[8]

Seeking closeness through sex and unconditional love from babies re-mains a viable option for poor teens. As Monique stated succinctly, "I'm safe, accepted, and comfortable with my man. . . . But my baby boy is all that no one else has been in my life. He will always love me. . . . [H]e has to."

I have shown that young women who either abstain from sex or wait until they are over sixteen or seventeen do so because they want to establish emotional closeness with their partner before physical inti-macy. They come from families in which sex is discussed but in which they are primarily expected to accomplish many other things academi-cally and professionally. In my study, sexuality and sex are not con-flated with identity in the same way that it can be for low-income teen-agers. More privileged teenagers have a broader range of behaviors that can symbolize attainment and adulthood than teens from low-SES backgrounds.

Adapting to one's social reality is as relevant to sexual behavior as it is to academic and career-related behavior.[9] These facts must be ac-counted for in sex education. Teenagers come from a variety of families and neighborhoods. Some have been raised to be comfortable with their sexuality. Their parents or guardians talk to them about sex and pregnancy. They do not experience pressure to defy their families' ex-pectations of them. The future is filled with some promise. Most important, they believe that they have some control over their future. Though having children may be an ultimate goal, it is not an immediate need.

Their lower-income peers, however, face a different set of expectations and attitudes. Parents raise them to be prepared for the reality of life in a poor neighborhood. Parents and mentors remind these teenagers that they need to work hard to be successful, that nothing can be expected without great effort. However, what the teenagers observe is that an education may not guarantee economic stability. Mortality surrounds them on a more regular basis. They are less likely to hold after-school jobs and are more likely to drop out of school. Survival is more dependent on "street smarts" than on schooling.[10] Feeling isolated from others and more suspicious, these young women view men as a source of pleasure, not companionship or life commitment. "'Slam-bam, thank you *man*' is what we all should be saying," observed one eighteen-year-old. Sex is a way to experience short-term intimacy without emotional ties.

Females are responsible for learning about, acquiring, and introducing contraceptive use in their intimate relationships. In other words, they are more likely to seek out methods that do not require male involvement directly. The chance that they will use condoms is therefore diminished. Early sexual experimentation is intercourse, not oral sex or other options, perhaps because other sexual activity connotes a different kind of intimacy than what young women seek. They express little concern for AIDS because risk, probability, and quality of life are concepts closely associated with having a future. If anything, children may represent the future, which again requires the rejection of all contraception or at least its irregular use. Delayed motherhood is of little consequence.[11]

Most teenagers know about AIDS and HIV.[12] They understand risk and the importance of condoms, yet inaccurately assess their own risk. I doubt that adults are very different from them. Condoms require conversation (i.e., negotiating with one's partner), and the participation of both partners. Condoms represent illness and AIDS rather than responsibility and commitment. Remember Helen, from chapter 6, who said that contraception "is bad news, because people will think you are sleeping around." And Ann, who saw condoms as "the quickest way to lose a boyfriend. He'll think you're sick, maybe with the AIDS disease." Given these kinds of sentiments, has AIDS education failed?

I believe it has. Although most young adults know about HIV, they do not understand how to identify their personal risk and are unwilling to do so. According to ARRM, knowledge is required to change behavior, but so are accurately identifying one's risk, committing to changing behaviors, and having the social support in doing so. It is unfair to expect youth to master skills most adults never acquire. Furthermore, given the different definitions and meanings attached to risk as outlined in this book, the failure of the current modes of education is understandable. All young adults must value themselves and believe in their ability to survive. Prevention programs must teach youth how to express intimacy, to develop trust, and to make the transition to adulthood.

We are now facing a new millennium in which people will face HIV and AIDS. This is a problem of global proportions. As internationally renown AIDS expert Jonathan Mann has argued, fundamentally AIDS is a human rights issue. Though devastating in its own right, this virus also highlights an array of social problems that young adults of all races have faced for years. I would be naive in arguing that the end of AIDS would hasten the end of poverty and inequality, but I do believe that the end of poverty and inequality would immediately diminish the new cases of HIV infection among young black women who are poor.

Appendix 1

Description of the Study

E thnography, field research, oral narrative collection, and related qualitative data collection methods have been popular tools for many social scientists. The legacy of these studies includes Elliot Lebow's *Tally's Corner*, Joyce Ladner's *Tomorrow's Tomorrow*, and Carol Stack's *All Our Kin*. Of note is that much of the ethnography collected by sociologists depicts the lives of groups and communities that are often misunderstood, misrepresented, or virtually invisible in social science inquiry. Teenagers, black men and women, poor families, single parents—these groups are traditionally the inspiration for such works. Although it can be argued that all of these groups are the target of large-scale quantitative projects, what remains to be proven is that these studies have consistently shed accurate light on their subjects. Sometimes the problem does not lie with the data but in the interpretation. Other times the flaw is in the way populations are identified and targeted, the way questions are constructed and asked.

In the more recent group of studies, some of which have been already mentioned in this book, these flaws are yet again identified. Furthermore, ethnographers are turning a critical eye to the works of other ethnographers. In *Slim's Table: Race, Respectability, and Masculinity* (1992), author and sociologist Mitch Duneier warns against the tendency to generalize stereotypes because they have been legitimized by social science research. He identifies this tendency in both the qualitative and the quantitative. Herbert J. Gans offers the same warning. All too often, he notes in *The War against the Poor*, social scientists' work is absorbed within the broader community and is accepted and perpetuated by the mass media with little question. The presumption is that numbers are never wrong—they represent objective fact: "the ethic of value-free social science and disinterested research also frees [social scientists] from thinking about the effects of both their research and their concepts" (56).

In an essay I contributed to Kim Marie Vaz's *Oral Narrative Research with Black Women: Collecting Treasures* (1997), I argue that ethnography is intended to shed light on populations that are simultaneously understudied and overstudied. By this I mean that communities are rendered invisible and are left silent by researchers who, though well intentioned, do not allow study participants to speak for themselves or to assume a more active role in the data collection process. I was motivated to encourage young black women to engage in what Janie Ward calls "truth telling" (Leadbeater and Way, 1997). Ethnography and the analysis of narratives facilitated truth telling.

My primary data source was a $2^1/2$ year field project conducted in the early 1990s. This approach enabled me to spend long periods of time with the fifty-three young women I came to know over the years. Some contact was in a classroom or during after-school meetings, at other times conversations occurred in more comfortable, familiar spaces. By becoming acquainted with the girls, I learned about their sexual behavior and decision-making process as well as the impact of their sexuality, poverty, and perception of motherhood and family on their intimate behaviors.

By using such a flexible method for primary data collection, I obtained a comprehensive picture of the experience and meaning of adolescence in the 1990s. My observations are intended to be illustrative of the kinds of issues faced by teenage black females today; they are not meant as typologies, archetypes, or generalizations. Instead, what I learned from these young women is that there are unifying principles in their experiences based on race, gender, and class; at the same time it is important to be mindful of the variation and uniqueness to be found among teenagers. The ultimate benefit of this method is that the young women had the opportunity to personalize—to make real—the epidemiological and demographic data concerning sexuality and sexual behavior among young people. Eventually, after some encouragement, they provided me with insights into adolescence that can only come from personal interaction.

In total, fifty-three young women provided the data I use in this book. These teenagers fall into two distinct groups. Forty-one young women comprised the core of my sample. I had regular contact with them throughout the course of the study. The majority of these young women—thirty-three—are black (see Table 1). Five Latinas and three white teenagers comprised the remaining eight participants in the group. The second group providing data for this project consisted of young women with whom my contact was less extensive. They occa-

TABLE 1
Racial Distribution of Sample

Race/Ethnicity	LEARN	Sistahs	Teen-Lead	The Exchange	Total
Black	7	5	10	11	33
Latina	2	1	2	0	5
White	0	1	0	2	3
Total	9	7	12	13	41

sionally participated in group interviews, and all of them completed a survey I developed. Seven women in this group are white, and five Latina.

Even though the number of case studies is relatively small, it was imperative that I build in some heterogeneity in my sample. Each organization or group attracted adolescents from different ethnic groups, age cohorts, neighborhoods, education levels, and socioeconomic statuses (SES). In deciding which programs to include in this study, I required that (1) they include participants who were representative of the background characteristics I wished to study and who lived in New Haven, (2) the administrators and outreach workers expressed interest in what I wanted to study, (3) education and outreach was a component of the program, and (4) the group met regularly.

I drew on four separate neighborhood organizations for participants. LEARN was an academic enrichment program that targeted youth of color. Participants attend urban public high schools where support resources often were limited. The purpose of LEARN is to capture teenagers with college aspirations and provide them with the encouragement to pursue their goals. There were fourteen participants, eleven of them female. Most of these teenagers had been involved in enrichment programs for years, and so they knew each other well. They were a vocal, opinionated group who enjoyed debating social issues. Their candor often surprised me. From this group I contacted nine young women. Seven were black, two of them Puerto Rican; all were juniors or seniors and ranged in age from fifteen to seventeen. Some lived in two-parent homes, while three lived with either one parent or a relative. All but one Puerto Rican woman reported having some level of sexual experience with boys, and they were more knowledgeable about contraceptives and STDs than many other teenagers I got to know. They were planning to go to college and had very precise expectations for their careers.

Teen-Lead and Sistahs were health oriented and had informal ties with health agencies in the community. Sistahs has provided young pregnant girls with counseling, parenting support, and educational skills development for about fifteen years. Each girl is referred to Sistahs by a case worker or guidance counselor. All but a handful are either black or Latina, and half are in school. These mothers-to-be talk about healthy living, sexual behavior, child care, and other issues that make them seem older than their years. But this image disappears rather quickly, and what emerges are young girls who are alternately excited and frightened by what lay ahead for them. The aim of this program is to provide a setting where these girls can share their hopes and fears and to introduce them to cultural and social resources that could benefit both them and their children. Five black teenagers and five Latinas eventually agreed to meet with me outside of the program. All but one lived with their parents, and two intended to marry the fathers of their children, but only once the babies were born.

In Teen-Lead, students from high school and junior high school are trained to be peer counselors inside their schools and to do street outreach with adult case workers. What is especially interesting about this program is that the participants have all been identified as "at risk" for dropping out of high school or for repeating a grade. The intention of the program counselors is to instill a strong sense of well-being in the future peer counselors through the training process. This after-school program meets year-round and includes many field trips to nearby city museums. Each participant is given some money as a reward for completing tasks on time and for attending consistently. This, along with the chance to spend time in a comfortable, safe haven, proved to be effective motivations for the participants.

Thirty active group members spend two to three hours a week talking, doing role-play, and receiving counseling. Teen-Lead has a familial, summer camp atmosphere, but these young adults are very aware of and responsive to the program director. Along with the coordinators, the director assumes the role of parent for these kids. Twelve young women met with me for this study. We spent time shopping, having lunch, or simply talking in the city's park.

The Exchange consisted of high school students who were interested in politics, culture, and activism. Parents were actively involved in this program. The goal was to provide a forum where these students could talk about their lives and ethnic, racial, cultural, and religious differences. The Exchange was virtually 50 percent white and 50 percent black. Some of the black participants had ties to Kenya, Jamaica, Antigua, the Dominican Republic, Korea, Russia, and Canada. Because of this variety, a popular topic of discussion was the pressure to be "culturally American" while retaining "native-born" identity. Even with this ethnic variety, participants always treated each other with respect.

Two program facilitators were the glue that kept this after-school group intact. One of them gave each student a hug at the beginning of meetings and kept up-to-date on the students' personal interests. Eight young women were very eager to be included in my study, and they quickly introduced me to an additional five teenagers.

As the story of The Exchange illustrates, I relied on a snowball sampling process. A few participants introduced me to their friends, who were then included in my sample; in turn, some of those friends introduced me to others. I conducted additional interviews with the directors of the programs with members who participated. The directors provided observations concerning their members as well as opinions on adolescent sexual behavior and effective educational and social support initiatives.

The age distribution of the sample was slightly skewed toward older teenagers; twenty-five were between sixteen and nineteen years old (only one was nineteen, a young mother), and the remaining sixteen were between thirteen and fifteen years old. This is accounted for by the number of young women from Teen-Lead and The Exchange who participated. The average age of participants was sixteen years old. In determining racial background, SES, and other measures, I depended on the young women's self-definition and to some extent supportive data I observed and collected from neighborhood/census tract data, case workers, teachers, counselors, and some parents.

Since I argue that perception of class and financial stability is relevant, I believed that it was important to account for the young women's self-definition in my analysis. Some difference is apparent between reported income and self-defined social class standing. What is particularly interesting is the extent to which the family income distribution found among the participants illustrates the racially mediated way income is distributed in many cities in the United States.

All of the participants coming from LEARN, Teen-Lead, and The Exchange were high school students. Fifty-six percent of teenage moth-

TABLE 2
Race and SES Characteristics of Sample

SES	Black	Latina	White	Total
Upper-middle	1	0	1	2
Middle	8	2	1	11
Working poor	15	1	0	16
Poor	9	2	1	12
Total	33	5	3	41

TABLE 3
Parents' Combined Yearly Income (Estimated) by Race

Income	Black	Latina	White	Total
$50,000 & over	0	0	2	2
$40,000–$49,999	1	0	0	1
$30,000–$39,999	3	0	0	3
$20,000–$29,999	4	1	0	5
$10,000–$19,999	16	1	1	18
$0–$9,999	8	3	0	11
Total	32	5	3	40*

*One respondent stated that she did not know her family's annual income.

ers participating in the "mothers teaching mothers" component of Sistahs were in high school. The remainder had not finished, but some expressed plans to resume high school or complete their GEDs. Most of the core sample had sex at least once (Table 4). Of this group, twenty more reported sexual activity at least once a month. Twenty-nine of the sexually active teenagers stated that they regularly contracept. Nineteen had used condoms during the past year. The seven young women who were pregnant or had given birth to at least one child were participants in Sistahs. Another four, from other programs, reported having been pregnant. These young women terminated their pregnancies. Most of the teenagers in the sample were sexually active (Table 5). Only six participants reported never experiencing any type of sexual activity, including oral sex. Four of the abstinent teens were black, one Latina, and one white.

I noted there was less racial variation in sexual behavior than some of my colleagues had expected. However, there is enough variation

TABLE 4
Rates of Sexual Activity, Contraceptive Use, and Pregnancy

	Black	Latina	White	Total
Sexually active	29	4	2	35
Ever pregnant	6	2	2	10
Do not contracept	5	1	0	6
Do contracept	24	3	2	29
Condoms	5	1	0	6
The pill	12	1	2	15
Sponge	7	0	0	7
Foam	1	0	0	1

TABLE 5
Sexual Activity by Race and SES

	Black	Latina	White	Total
Upper-middle-class	1	0	1	2
Middle-class	5	1	0	6
Working poor	14	1	0	15
Poor	9	2	1	12
Total	29	4	2	35

by SES to merit a discussion of social class as a mediating factor in reproductive behavior, sexuality, and risk. This point could be elaborated in future research by generating a larger heterogeneous sample in terms of race, ethnicity, and SES.

Appendix 2

HIV- and AIDS-Related Resources

onsidering the rapid growth in available information, the following list cannot be exhaustive. Rather, it represents a cross-section of the various sources and kinds of information available to the public. Reference to these sources should not be construed as an endorsement or validation of the quality or accuracy of what they provide.

Federal Agencies

Centers for Disease Control National AIDS Clearinghouse
P.O. Box 6003
Rockville, Md. 20849-6003
General information: 1-800-458-5231; fax, 1-800-458-5231
Clinical trials: 1-800-TRIALS-A
Treatment information: 1-800-HIV-0440
E-mail: aidsinfo@cdcnac.org
Web site: http://www.cdcnac.org
The CDC clearinghouse offers a variety of resources, including educational materials for different target groups such as adolescents and women. Materials include books, brochures, catalogs, posters, and videos. Some material is free, and many are available in Spanish.

National Institutes of Health (NIH) Office of AIDS Research
Building 31, Room 4C06
Bethesda, Md. 20892
General information: 301-402-3555; fax, 301-496-4843

State and Local Agencies

The Department of Health in virtually every state has a division or agency devoted to AIDS and HIV research, prevention, and treatment. All numbers are for in-state calls.

State Hot Lines:

Alabama: 1-800-228-0469
Alaska: 1-800-478-2437
Arizona: 1-800-334-1540
Arkansas: 1-800-364-2437
California
   Southern California: 1-800-992-2437
   Los Angeles: 1-213-876-2437
   Northern California: 1-800-367-2437
   Filipino: 1-800-345-AIDS
Colorado: 1-800-252-2437
Connecticut: 1-800-203-1234
Delaware: 1-800-422-0429
District of Columbia: 1-800-322-7432
Florida: 1-800-352-AIDS (English), 1-800-545-SIDA (Spanish),
   1-800-243-7101 (Haitian Creole)
Georgia: 1-800-551-2728
Hawaii: 1-800-321-1555
Idaho: 1-800-677-2437
Illinois: 1-800-243-2437
Indiana: 1-800-843-2437
Iowa: 1-800-445-2437
Kansas: 1-800-232-0040
Kentucky: 1-800-840-2865
Louisiana: 1-800-992-4379
Maine: 1-800-851-2437
Maryland: 1-800-638-6252 (bilingual), 1-800-322-7432 (metro D.C. and
   Virginia area)
Massachusetts: 1-800-235-2331
Michigan: 1-800-872-2437, 1-800-750-TEEN (teen line)
Minnesota: 1-800-248-2437
Mississippi: 1-800-826-2961
Missouri: 1-800-533-2437
Montana: 1-800-233-6668
Nebraska: 1-800-782-2437
Nevada: 1-800-842-2437

New Hampshire: 1-800-752-2437
New Jersey: 1-800-624-2377
New Mexico: 1-800-545-2437
New York: 1-800-541-2437, 1-800-233-7432 (Spanish)
North Dakota: 1-800-472-2180
Ohio: 1-800-332-2437
Oregon: 1-800-777-2437
Pennsylvania: 1-800-662-6080
Puerto Rico: 1-800-981-5721
Rhode Island: 1-800-726-3010, 1-800-442-7432 (Spanish)
South Carolina: 1-800-322-2437
South Dakota: 1-800-592-1861
Tennessee: 1-800-525-AIDS
Texas: 1-800-299-2437
Utah: 1-800-366-2437
Vermont: 1-800-882-2437
Virgin Islands: 1-809-773-2437
Virginia: 1-800-533-4148, 1-800-322-7432 (Spanish)
Washington: 1-800-272-2437
West Virginia: 1-800-642-8244
Wisconsin: 1-800-334-2437
Wyoming: 1-800-327-3577

City *AIDS Projects*
Most of these are based in cities around the country. The organizations are nonprofit service providers for people affected by either AIDS or HIV.

AIDS Advocacy Organizations and Hot Lines

The local Yellow Pages usually has a listing for an information hot line that offers confidential counseling and information, and facilitates testing.

AIDS Clinical Trials Information Service: 1-800-TRIALS-A
American Foundation for AIDS Research (AMFAR): 1-212-682-7440
American Social Health Association: 1-919-361-8400
The Committee of Ten Thousand (grass-roots advocacy group for people who contracted HIV from blood products): 1-800-488-COTT (2688) or 1-202-543-0988
The Condom Resource Center: 1-510-891-0455

HIV/AIDS Treatment Information Service: 1-800-448-0440,
    1-800-243-7012 (TDD)
Minority AIDS Project: 1-213-936-4949
Minority Task Force on AIDS: 1-212-870-2691
National AIDS Hot Line: 1-800-342-AIDS
National Association of People with AIDS: 1-202-898-0414
National Minority AIDS Council: 1-800-559-4145
National Native American AIDS Prevention Center: 1-800-293-2437
National Resource Center on Women and AIDS: 1-202-872-1770
Pediatric AIDS Foundation: 1-310-395-9051
Project Inform Hot Line: 1-800-822-7422
SisterLove, Inc.: 1-404-753-7733
Women Alive: 1-800-554-4876
Women Organized to Respond to Life-Threatening Diseases (WORLD):
    1-510-658-6930
Women's AIDS Network: 1-415-621-4160

Internet Sites

Many Web sites are devoted solely to AIDS and HIV issues, as well
as many others featuring relevant information. Since the Internet is
unregulated, variety in the kinds of information offered, the intended
audience, and so on, is available. Consider these among the many tools
available for investigation.

Web Sites

AIDS Research Information Center (ARIC): http: //www.critpath.
    org/aric/
A Web site intended for laypeople, ARIC includes a medical information service and a medical inquiry service. It also provides access to a
variety of publications including the ARIC AIDS medicine glossary,
and a newsletter.

AIDS Clinical Trials Information Service (ACTIS): http://
    www.actis.org/
This site provides information on HIV/AIDS clinical trials and on results. Links to other sites.

AIDS Coalition to Unleash Power (ACT-UP): http://
    www.actupny.org/

This New York–based branch of the organization provides support and referral for clients throughout the United States. The Web site offers a variety of instructional information.

AIDS Treatment Information Service (ATIS): http://www.hivatis.org/
Contact: atis@cdcnac.aspensys.com
Information is available here about federally approved treatments for HIV infection and links to other treatment-related sites.

AIDS Virtual Library: http://planetq.com/aidsvl/index.html/
Updated regularly, this site offers information on conferences, archives, organizations, statistical reports, on-line periodicals, and relevant organizations.

Center For AIDS Research (CFAR): http://
    mediswww.meds.cwrv.edu/cfar/default.html/
Case Western Reserve University is host to one of the eleven CFARs around the nation. The center connects research with community-based education and support facilities. It provides a few links to other Web sites that may be mostly oriented toward research and clinical trials.

Center for Disease Control (CDC) publications and services page:
    http://www.cdc.gov/ publication.htm/
This site includes summary reports of rates of infection/incidence and prevention guidelines. It also provides back issues of the *HIV/AIDS Surveillance Report* in ASCII format and PDF format.

Department of Health and Human Services: http://
    www.os.dhhs.gov/
From this site you can access the CDC (Centers for Disease Control), FDA (Federal Drug Administration), NIH (National Institutes of Health), SAMHSA (Substance Abuse and Mental Health Services Administration), ACF (Administration for Children and Families), as well as many other government agencies.

Family AIDS Network: http://www.aidsquilt.org and http://
    www.aidsquilt.org/aidsinfo

The former site provides information on the AIDS quilt; the latter one offers general AIDS information.

FedWorld: http://www.fedworld.gov/
This is probably one of the most "linked" federal government sites. It can connect you to at least 130 government bulletin boards. Information is organized by subject and can be sorted by keywords.

Harvard University AIDS Institute: gopher://gopher.harvard.edu.70/
   00/.vine/providers/aids_institute/aids
This site offers research information and links to other research sites.

HIV/AIDS: gopher://riceinfo.rice.edu:70/11/Safety/HealthInfo/hiv
This site presents information on a study of women and HIV, including an analysis of risk factors. Contact Prentice Riddle: riddle@rice.edu

JAMA (Journal of the American Medical Association) HIV/AIDS
   Information Center: http://www.ama-assn.org/special/hiv/
   hivhome.htm/
An archive of various resources for health care providers and the general public, this site includes clinical updates, news, and other kinds of information. It also posts articles from leading medical journals and federal health agencies.

National Association of People With AIDS (NAPWA): http://
   www.thecure.org/
Interested visitors also can call 1-800-786-1693.

National Institutes of Allergy and Infectious Diseases (NIAID): http://
   www.niaid.nih.gov/ default.htm#abt
Materials here are divided into four categories: About NIAID, Information (news, upcoming events, publications), Research Activities, and Opportunities (clinical trials, employment, grants).

National Library of Medicine (NLM): http://www.nlm.nih.gov/
This is a Web site representing information from NIH, and the Depart-

ment of Health and Human Services, among others. Sites include news items, databases, NLM publications, research programs, and grants.

Office of AIDS and Special Health Issues (OASHI): http://
www.fda.gov/ (click on AIDS)
This office is part of the Food and Drug Administration (FDA).

Project Inform: http://www.projinf.org/
This site offers some information in Spanish and English.

The Safer Sex Page: http://www.safersex.org/
Many links to other sites are available through this page. Most information is meant for educational purposes, such as defining safer sex and demonstrating the effective uses of barrier contraception. Some information involves graphics and thus is visually explicit.

SisterLove Home Page: http://hidwater.com/sisterlove/
This Web page provides organizational information and contact sources. A full description is listed under "Organizations."

Stop AIDS Project: http://www.stopaids.org/
This site is devoted primarily to gay men in the San Francisco area.

United Nations Program on HIV/AIDS (UNAIDS): http://
gpawww.who.ch/index.html/
This organization focuses on advocacy, policy development, technical support, and other services. The Web site is devoted to the question of AIDS/HIV research, intervention, incidence, and clinical care on a global level. It provides these resources by linking viewers with other UN-affiliated organizations' sites.

University of Michigan's Guide to Women's Health Issues:
http://asa.ugl.lib.umich.edu/chdocs/womenhealth/
womens_health.html/
This site provides links to other Internet resources concerning women's health.

Women and HIV Infection:
  http://www.cmpharm,ucsf.edu/~troyer/safesex/vanews/
  vanewswomen.html/
This site provides articles about women and HIV/AIDS from the Virginia AIDS Information Newsletter.

Electronic Bulletin Boards

AEGIS_World_HQ
Sister Mary Elizabeth, Sisters of St. Elizabeth of Hungary, P.O. Box 184,
  San Juan Capistrano, Calif. 92693-0184
Data line: 1-714-248-2836
The AIDS Education and Global Information System is a network of bulletin boards concerned with HIV-related issues. It includes clippings and files that may be downloaded. Contact Sister Mary Elizabeth for software or further information.

CDC NAC Online
Rockville, Md.
Data line: 1-800-851-5231
The National AIDS Clearinghouse (NAC) network offers information for nonprofit AIDS-related organizations. Covers education, testing, legislation, and upcoming events. It provides access to interactive bulletin board forums and a clipping service.

Women's Wire
By subscription only: call 1-415-615-8989 or E-mail subscribe@wwire.net. Include your name, phone number, address, type of computer, and system.
This bulletin board provides information on women from news sources, government, women's organizations, and from subscribers themselves.

Research Centers and Institutes

Some institutes are affiliated with research universities that are devoted to the study of HIV and AIDS around the United States. Many are listed in Internet sites. Otherwise, check with the nearest university for information on newsletters, conferences, symposia, and published works they may distribute.

Notes

Introduction

1. I use the term *black* rather than *African-American* throughout this book. Even so, I must clarify what I see as some important distinctions. Debate has continued over the social, political, and ideological meaning of using black versus African-American. In my opinion, each term refers to a different cohort of color. African-American excludes blacks who come from the Caribbean, Central and South America, Haiti, and the rest of the Diaspora. It is a category that often ignores the cultural and historical differences that exist among all people of African descent. Unfortunately, the range of cultural distinctions among the young women represented in this project cannot be addressed in their entirety.

2. Further details about New Haven and teenagers are in Chapter 2 and Appendix 1.

Chapter 1

1. Unprotected sex allows for bodily contact with semen (sperm), vaginal secretions, and blood. These substances can carry HIV.

2. Once researchers recognized that drugs made with any component of human blood could transmit HIV, such as anticoagulants for hemophiliacs, they initiated rigorous testing of all blood used and altered the drug production process. Since 1985, all blood—meaning what is used for transfusions as well as what is used for these drugs—has been tested for HIV. Additionally, organs used for transplants are tested for HIV.

3. The probability of prenatal transmission (the passage of HIV to a fetus during pregnancy or childbirth) could be 15 to 45 percent (Women Organized to Respond to Life-Threatening Diseases, September 1991).

4. New York State Department of Health, "Overview of HIV Infection and AIDS," in *Participant's Manual* (New York: New York State AIDS Institute, 1991).

5. See William A. Blattner, "HIV Epidemiology: Past, Present, and Future," *FASEB Journal* 5 (1990): 2340–48; Hung Fan, Ross F. Conner, and Luis P. Villarreal, *AIDS: Science and Society* (Sudbury, Mass: Jones & Bartlet, 1998), 68–71.

6. In the early years of the AIDS epidemic, what she experienced would have been called early AIDS–related complex (ARC) and then severe ARC—full-blown AIDS.

7. Fan et al., *AIDS*, 105–9.

8. *Morbidity and Mortality Weekly Report* (MMWR) 46, no. 8, mmwr-asc@listserv.cdc.gov, (February 28, 1997).

9. Centers for Disease Control (CDC), *HIV/AIDS Surveillance*, http://www.cdc.gov/ (March 1998).

10. CDC, *HIV/AIDS*.

11. "The window" refers to the period of time between contracting HIV and being tested HIV +. It is an estimate based on the period in which the majority of people who carry the virus are likely to test HIV-positive. The interval between contracting HIV and being diagnosed with AIDS depends in part on behavioral factors, including diet, exercise, drug treatment, and stress reduction.

12. Connecticut Department of Public Health and Addiction Services (DPHAS), *AIDS in Connecticut: Annual Surveillance Report, December 31, 1993* (Hartford: AIDS Section, DPHAS, 1994).

13. Connecticut Department of Public Health (DPH), *AIDS in Connecticut: Annual Surveillance Report, December 31, 1996* (Hartford: AIDS Epidemiology Program—Infectious Diseases Division, DPH, 1997).

14. DPHAS, *AIDS in Connecticut*, 1–4.

15. DPH, *AIDS in Connecticut*, 15.

16. Ronald Bayer, "AIDS and the Future of Reproductive Freedom," *Milbank Quarterly* 68 Suppl., no. 2 (1990): 179–204; Marshall H. Becker and Jill G. Joseph, "AIDS and Behavior Change to Reduce Risk: A Review," *American Journal of Public Health* 78, no. 4 (1988): 394–410; Howard B. Kaplan, Carol A. Bailey, and William Simon, "The Sociological Study of AIDS: A Critical Review of the Literature and Suggested Research Agenda," *Journal of Health and Social Behavior* 28 (1987): 140–57.

17. Bayer, "AIDS and the Future"; Carol Levine, "AIDS and Changing Concepts of Family," *Milbank Quarterly* 68 Suppl., no. 1 (1990): 33–57; Carola Marte and Kathryn Anastos, "Women—The Missing Persons in the AIDS Epidemic (Part II)," *Health/Pac Bulletin* (Spring 1990): 11–18.

18. Rosalind T. Harrison Chirimuuta and Richard C. Chirimuuta, "AIDS from Africa: A Case of Racism vs. Science?" in *AIDS in Africa and the Caribbean*, ed. George C. Bond, John Kreniske, Ida Susser, and Joan Vincent (Boulder, Colo.: Westview, 1997), 165–80.

19. The debate over women infecting others is commonly grounded in the perception of them as "vectors of transmission" whose sexual behavior and reproductive rights have to be controlled in the best interests of the children (see Bayer 1990; Oakley 1980; Richie 1990).

20. Joseph P. Allen, Susan Philliber, and Nancy Hoggson, "School Based Pre-

vention of Teenage Pregnancy and School Dropout: Process Evaluation of National Replication of Teen Outreach Programs," *American Journal of Community Psychology* 18, no. 4 (1990): 505–24; Arline Geronimus, "Teenage Childbearing and Social and Reproductive Disadvantage: The Evolution of Complex Questions and the Demise of Simple Answers," *Family Relations* 40 (1991): 463–71; Lorraine P. Mayfield, "Early Parenthood among Low–Income Girls," in *The Black Family*, ed. Robert Staples (Belmont, Calif.: Wadsworth, 1986).

21. Many resources are available through the National AIDS Information Clearinghouse, which is affiliated with the CDC. These, and others, are listed in Appendix 2.

22. Joyce Ladner, *Tomorrow's Tomorrow: The Black Woman* (New York: Doubleday, 1995); Carol B. Stack, *All Our Kin: Strategies for Survival in a Black Community* (New York: Harper & Row, 1974); Carol B. Stack and Linda M. Burton, "Kinscripts: Reflections on Family, Generation, and Culture," in *Mothering: Ideology, Experience, and Agency*, ed. Evelyn Nakano Glenn, Grace Chang, and Linda Rennie Forcey (New York: Routledge, 1994).

23. Daniel Patrick Moynihan, *The Negro Family: The Case for National Action* (Washington, D.C.: Office of Policy Planning and Research, U.S. Department of Labor, 1965); Charles Murray, *Losing Ground: American Social Policy 1950–1980* (New York: Basic Books, 1995); See Solinger (1994) for a description of a number of studies sponsored by the U.S. government that reflected this image of black families and culture.

24. Angela Y. Davis, *Women, Culture, and Politics* (New York: Vintage Books, 1990); Constance Nathanson, *Dangerous Passage: The Social Control of Sexuality in Women's Adolescence* (Philadelphia: Temple University Press, 1991); Margaret K. Rosenheim and Mark F. Testa, eds., *Early Parenthood and Coming of Age in the 1990s* (New Brunswick, N.J.: Rutgers University Press, 1992).

Chapter 2

1. Deborah Tolman, "Adolescent Girls' Sexuality: Debunking the Myth of the Urban Girl," in *Urban Girls: Resisting Stereotypes, Creating Identities*, ed. Leadbeater and Way (New York: New York University Press, 1996), 255.

2. See Patricia Hill Collins, *Black Feminist Thought* (Boston: Unwin Hyman, 1990); Calvin C. Hernton, *Sex and Racism in America* (New York: Anchor Books, 1965/1992).

3. See Jill Quadagno, *The Color of Welfare* (New York: Oxford University Press, 1994).

4. James E. Rosenbaum and Susan J. Popkin, "Employment and Earnings of Low-Income Blacks Who Move to Middle Class Suburbs," in *The Urban Underclass*, ed. Christopher Jencks and Paul E. Peterson, (Washington, D.C.: Brookings Institution, 1991), 343.

5. Dionne J. Jones and Stanley F. Battle, eds., *Teenage Pregnancy: Developmental Strategies for Change in the Twenty First Century* (New Brunswick, N.J.: Transaction, 1990), 20.

6. Sol Gordon and Jane F. Gilgun, "Adolescent Sexuality," in *Handbook of Adolescent Psychology*, ed. Vincent Van Hasselt and Michael Herson (New York: Pergamon, 1987), 154.

7. Davis, *Women*, 75.

8. Robert Staples and Leanor Boulin Johnson, *Black Families at the Crossroads: Challenges and Prospects* (San Francisco: Jossey-Bass, 1993).

9. Staples, ed., *The Black Family*; 230–31; italics have been added.

10. This is the result of industrial relocation from urban areas and a shift from manufacturing to technical service-oriented industries, which require more preparatory training for entry-level jobs.

11. Jones and Battle, eds., *Teenage Pregnancy*, 18.

12. Vonnie McLoyd and Debra M. Hernandez Jozefowicz, "Sizing Up Their Future: Predictors of African American Adolescent Females' Expectancies about Their Economic Fortunes and Family Life Courses," in *Urban Girls*, ed. Leadbeater and Way, 355–79.

13. Elijah Anderson, *Streetwise: Race, Class and Change in an Urban City* (Chicago: University of Chicago Press, 1990), 72–73.

14. Connecticut Economic Information System (CEIS), http://www.state.ct.us/ecd/research/ceis/ (March 1998).

15. New Haven Census, "Income and Poverty Status in 1989," New Haven 1990, CPH–L–83, Table 3 http://www.statlab.stat.yale.edu/cityroom/NHOL.html/.

16. CEIS, March 1998.

17. Leadership, Education, and Athletics in Partnership (LEAP), Summer 1997; http://www.leap.yale.edu.

18. CEIS, March 1998.

19. LEAP, Summer 1997.

20. LEAP, Summer 1997.

21. Unfortunately, statistics were not available from the police department. According to a data analyst, statistics are only kept for a month. Therefore, longitudinal analyses are not available to the public.

22. All names have been changed to protect the participants' privacy.

23. James Diego Vigil, "Gangs, Social Control, and Ethnicity: Ways to Redirect," in *Identity and Inner City Youth: Beyond Ethnicity and Gender*, ed. Shirley Brice Heath and Milbrey McLaughlin (New York: Teachers College Press, 1993), 94–119.

24. LEAP, Summer 1997.

25. Kathleen Maguire and Ann L. Pastore, eds., *Sourcebook of Criminal Justice Statistics 1996* (Washington, D.C.: U.S. Department of Justice, Bureau of Justice Statistics, 1997), 209, 213.

26. Milbrey McLaughlin, "Embedded Identities: Enabling Balance in Urban Contexts," in *Identity and Inner City Youth*, Heath and McLaughlin, 36–68.

27. Major businesses have closed stores located in New Haven. In addition, longtime businesses continue to close. Since January 1996, part of the downtown area has become a virtual ghost town.

28. Susan Vance, R.N., M.P.H., Connecticut State Department of Public

Health—AIDS Epidemiology Program, personal correspondence on March 9, 1998.

29. See Appendix 1 for additional information on participants.

Chapter 3

1. Victor Gecas, "Contexts of Socialization," in *Social Psychology: Sociological Perspectives*, ed. Morris Rosenberg and Ralph Turner (New York: Basic Books, 1981), 165–99; Naomi Ruth Harris, "Teen Pregnancy: An Examination of Related Factors," unpublished thesis, Yale University School of Medicine, 1991; Levine, "AIDS and Changing Concepts"; Anita C. Washington, "A Cultural and Historical Perspective on Pregnancy-Related Activity among U.S. Teenagers," *Journal of Black Psychology* 9, no. 1 (1982): 1–28.

2. Catherine G. Ansuini, Robert Woite, and Julianna Fiddler Woite, "The Source, Accuracy, and Impact of Initial Sexuality Information on Lifetime Wellness," *Adolescence* 31, no. 122 (1996): 287.

3. Peggy Giordano, Stephen Cernkovich, and Alfred DeMaris, "The Family and Peer Relations of Black Adolescents," *Journal of Marriage and the Family* 55 (1993): 278.

4. Robert Taylor, Linda M. Chatters, M. Belinda Tucker, and Edith Lewis, "Development in Research on Black Families," *Journal of Marriage and the Family* 52 (1990): 995.

5. Ana Mari Cauce, Yumi Hiraga, Diane Graves, Nancy Gonzales, Kimberly Ryan–Finn, and Kwai Grove, "African American Mothers and Their Adolescent Daughters: Closeness, Conflict, and Control," in *Urban Girls: Resisting Stereotypes, Creating Identities*, ed. Leadbeater and Way, 100–16.

6. Jencks and Peterson, eds., *The Urban Underclass*, 384.

7. Renata Forste and Tim B. Heaton, "Initiation of Sexual Activity among Female Adolescents," *Youth and Society* 19, no. 3 (1988), 250–68.

8. Felissa Cohen and Jerry Durham, *Women, Children, and HIV/AIDS* (New York: Springer, 1993); Douglas Feldman, *Culture and AIDS* (New York: Praeger, 1990).

9. Shirley Vining Brown, "Premarital Sexual Permissiveness among Black Adolescent Females," *Social Psychology Quarterly* 48, no. 4 (1985), 381–87; Victor De La Cancela, "Minority AIDS Prevention: Moving beyond Cultural Perspectives towards Sociopolitical Empowerment," *AIDS Education and Prevention* 1, no. 2 (1989), 141–53; Ralph J. DiClemente, "Predictors of HIV-Preventive Sexual Behavior in a High-Risk Adolescent Population: Influence of Perceived Peer Norms and Sexual Communication on Incarcerated Adolescents' Consistent Use of Condoms," *Society for Adolescent Medicine* 12 (1991): 385–90.

10. Greer Litton Fox, "The Family's Role in Adolescent Sexual Behavior," in *Teenage Pregnancy in a Family Context*, ed. T. Ooms (Philadelphia: Temple University Press, 1981).

11. See Robert Merton, *Social Theory and Social Structure* (New York: Free Press, 1968), for Merton's use of functional analysis. Innovators are individuals

who seek out commonly held social goals but do not have access to traditional means for doing so. Thus, they use alternate means.

12. Gecas, "Contexts"; Washington, "A Cultural and Historical Perspective."

13. Levine, "AIDS and Changing Concepts."

14. Harris, "Teen Pregnancy," 29.

15. Gecas, "Contexts," 169.

16. Robert B. Cairns and Beverly D. Cairns, *Lifelines and Risks: Pathways of Youth in Our Time* (Cambridge: Cambridge University Press, 1994).

17. Jeanne Brooks-Gunn and Frank Furstenberg, Jr., "Coming of Age in the Era of AIDS: Puberty, Sexuality, and Contraception," *The Milbank Quarterly* 68 Suppl. (1990): 59–84; Bruce Hare, "African-American Youth at Risk," in *Teenage Pregnancy*, ed. Jones and Battle; Brent C. Miller, Roger B. Christensen, and Terrance O. Olson, "Adolescent Self-Esteem in Relation to Sexual Attitudes and Behavior," *Youth and Society* 19, no. 1 (1987): 93–111.

18. Elliot Aronson, Carrie Fried, and Jeff Stone, "Overcoming Denial and Increasing the Intention to Use Condoms through Induction of Hypocrisy," *American Journal of Public Health* 81, no. 12 (1991): 1636–38; DiClemente, "Predictors."

19. Niobe Way, "Between Experiences of Betrayal and Desire: Close Friendships among Urban Adolescents," in *Urban Girls*, ed. Leadbeater and Way, 173–192.

20. In general, research on peer pressure and role models assumes that teenagers' behavior is solely affected by their friends' opinions and expectations. We often argue that peer pressure only exists in adolescence; we fail to recognize that teenagers, like any age group, have varying thresholds of resistance to their friends' influence.

21. Greg J. Duncan and Saul D. Hoffman, "Teenage Underclass Behavior and Subsequent Poverty: Have the Rules Changed?" in *The Urban Underclass*, ed. Jencks and Peterson, 155–74; Tolman, "Adolescent Girls' Sexuality."

22. Eli Ginzberg, Howard S. Berliner, and Miriam Ostow, *Young People at Risk: Is Prevention Possible?* (Boulder, Colo.: Westview, 1988); Brent C. Miller and Kristin Moore and Rosenthal, "Adolescent Sexual Behavior, Pregnancy, and Parenting: Research through the 1980's," *Journal of Marriage and the Family* 52 (1990): 1025–44.

23. Duncan and Hoffman, "Teenage Underclass Behavior."

24. See Martha M. Dore and Ana O. Dumois, "Cultural Differences in the Meaning of Adolescent Pregnancy," *Families in Society* (February 1990): 93–101. Their interpretation of findings is curious. Claiming that there is a racial-ethnic distinction in susceptibility to peer pressure is a causal argument that Dore and Dumois did not conclusively show with their data. My findings indicate that responsiveness to peer pressure may be determined by the importance placed on maintaining social status.

25. In fact, I would argue that often the concept of peer pressure is used as a metaphor describing the way teenagers perceive of and respond to social norms. As such, it refers to a series of behavioral responses that extend beyond a passive response to the expectations of peers.

26. Anderson, *Streetwise*.

27. Cairns and Cairns, *Lifelines*.

28. Anderson, *Streetwise*; Beth Richie, "AIDS in Living Color," in *The Black Women's Health Book*, ed. Evelyn White (Seattle: Seal, 1990), 182–86; Washington, "A Cultural and Historical Perspective."

Chapter 4

1. Elise Jones, Jacqueline D. Forrest, Noreen Goldman, Stanley Henshaw, Richard Lincoln, Jeannie Rosoff, Charles Westoff, and Diedre Wulf, *Teenage Pregnancy in Industrialized Countries* (New Haven, Conn.: Yale University Press, 1986).

2. A number of authors in Leadbeater and Way, eds., *Urban Girls* make note of this silence in the literature as does Judith Musick in *Young, Poor and Pregnant: The Psychology of Teenage Motherhood* (New Haven, Conn.: Yale University Press, 1993).

3. Cairns and Cairns, *Lifelines*, focuses on life course and risk, but there is little on the process of relationship development. *Sex and Pregnancy in Adolescence* (Thousand Oaks, Calif.: Sage, 1981) by Melvin Zelnik, John Kantner, and Kathleen Ford is a landmark study and thus widely cited. However, it focuses on the analysis of race and class trends in sexual activity, contraceptive use, and pregnancy without effectively accounting for the process leading up to these outcomes. Both Carol Stack's *All Our Kin* (1974) and Joyce Ladner's *Tomorrow's Tomorrow* (1995) are two additional influential publications, yet the era they capture is not the same as the world in which young women of the 1990s live.

Sharon Thompson's *Going All the Way: Teenage Girls' Tales of Sex, Romance, and Pregnancy* (New York: Hill & Wang, 1995) and Leon Dash's *When Children Want Children* (New York: Morrow, 1989) are both powerful contemporary accounts that deal with race and class, yet neither author is a sociologist.

4. Developmental theory in both psychology and social psychology stress the importance of mimicry and games in childhood. Assuming different perspectives and roles enables children to understand what behaviors are appropriate in a given situation and how others will respond. What this indicates is that young children will reflect the behaviors they observe and to some extent what they hear. So if an adult expresses a progressive view of gender roles yet behaves very traditionally, her child might simply copy the behavior and remain unaware of her mother's ideological views regarding gender roles.

5. Diane Scott-Jones and Anne B. White, "Correlates of Sexual Activity in Early Adolescence," *Journal of Early Adolescence* 10, no. 2 (1990): 224.

6. Anderson, *Streetwise*, 113.

7. See essays in Rosenheim and Testa, eds., *Early Parenthood*, and Thompson, *Going All the Way*, for additional discussion of the relationship between social class and gender roles. I also observe how this relation between class and gender influences perceptions of sexual violence in "In the Name of Love

and Survival: Interpretations of Sexual Violence among Young Black American Women," in *Spoils of War: Women of Color, Cultures, and Revolutions*, ed. T. Denean Sharpley-Whiting and Renée T. White (Lanham, Md.: Rowman & Littlefield, 1997), 27–45.

8. Ladner, *Tomorrow's Tomorrow*, 181–82.

9. Diane Mitsch Bush and Roberta G. Simmons, "Socialization Patterns over the Life-Course," in *Social Psychology: Sociological Perspectives*, ed. Morris Rosenberg and Ralph Turner (New York: Basic Books, 1981), 133–64.

10. See chapter 3, note 11, for further discussion of innovation.

11. Linda Lindsey, *Gender Roles: A Sociological Perspective* (Upper Saddle River, N.J.: Prentice Hall, 1997); Susan Moore and Doreen Rosenthal, *Sexuality in Adolescence* (New York: Routledge, 1993).

12. Margaret R. Weeks, Jean Schensul, Sunya S. Williams, Merrill Singer, and Maryland Grier, "AIDS Prevention for African-American and Latina Women: Building Culturally and Gender-Appropriate Intervention," *AIDS Education and Prevention* 7, no. 3 (1995): 251–63.

13. Hortensia Amaro, "Love, Sex, and Power: Considering Women's Realities in HIV Prevention," *American Psychologist* 50, no. 6 (1995): 437–47; Scott-Jones and White, "Correlates."

14. Michelle Fine, "Sexuality, Schooling and Adolescent Females: The Missing Discourse of Desire," *Harvard Educational Review* 58, no. 1 (1988): 32.

15. White, "In the Name of Love."

16. Amaro, "Love."

17. Moore and Rosenthal, *Sexuality*; Thompson, *Going All the Way*.

18. Amaro, "Love"; Ladner, *Tomorrow's Tomorrow*.

19. See chapter 5 for a detailed discussion of these studies.

20. Parts of this conversation are paraphrased.

21. White, "In the Name of Love."

22. Ladner, *Tomorrow's Tomorrow*.

23. Moore and Rosenthal, *Sexuality*, 6.

Chapter 5

1. Kristin Luker, *Dubious Conceptions: The Politics of Teenage Pregnancy* (Cambridge, Mass: Harvard University Press, 1997); Zelnik et al., *Sex and Pregnancy*.

2. Rickie Solinger, "Race and 'Value': Black and White Illegitimate Babies, 1945–1965," in *Mothering*, ed. Glenn, Chang, and Forcey (New York: Routlege, 1994).

3. See, for example, Collins, *Black Feminist Thought*, and Hernton, *Sex and Racism*, who offer critiques of this pseudo–scientific argument.

4. Brooks-Gunn and Furstenberg, "Coming of Age"; Fox, "The Family's Role."

5. Amaro, "Love"; Arline Geronimus, "Teenage Childbearing and Social

Disadvantage: Unprotected Discourse," *Family Relations* 41 (1992): 244–48; Staples, *The Black Family*; Washington, "A Cultural and Historical Perspective."

6. Harris, "Teen Pregnancy"; George Lowenstein and Frank Furstenberg, "Is Teenage Sexual Behavior Rational?" *Journal of Applied Social Psychology* 21, no. 12 (1991): 957–86.

7. Peter Edelman and Joyce Ladner, *Adolescence and Poverty: Challenge for the 1990s* (Washington, D.C.: Center for National Policy Press, 1991); Washington, "A Cultural and Historical Perspective."

8. Levine, "AIDS and Changing Concepts," 34.

9. Hugh Klein, "Adolescence, Youth and Young Adulthood: Rethinking Current Conceptualizations of Life Stage," *Youth and Society* 21, no. 4 (1990), 456–57.

10. Harris, "Teen Pregnancy"; Lowenstein and Furstenberg, "Is Teenage Sexual Behavior Rational?"; Staples, *The Black Family*.

11. Hare, "African-American Youth"; Harris, "Teen Pregnancy."

12. Washington, "A Cultural and Historical Perspective."

13. Joy Dryfoos, *Adolescents at Risk: Prevalence and Prevention* (New York: Oxford University Press, 1990); Priscilla Koyle, Fay Carter, Larry C. Jensen, Joe Olsen, and Bert Cundick, "Comparison of Sexual Behaviors among Adolescents Having an Early, Middle and Late First Intercourse Experience," *Youth and Society* 20, no. 4 (1989): 461–76.

14. Brown, "Premarital Sexual Permissiveness"; Lowenstein and Furstenberg, "Is Teenage Sexual Behavior Rational?"; John M. Wallace and Jerald Bachman, "Explaining Racial/Ethnic Differences in Adolescent Drug Use: The Impact of Background and Lifestyle," *Social Problems* 38, no. 3 (1991): 333–57.

15. Geronimus, "Teenage Childbearing," 469.

16. Brown, "Premarital Sexual Permissiveness."

17. Steven P. Schinke, Gilbert Botvin, Mario A. Orlandi, Robert F. Schilling, and Adam N. Gordon, "African-American and Hispanic-American Adolescents, HIV Infection and Preventative Intervention," *AIDS Education and Prevention* 2, no. 4: 305–12.

18. Forste and Heaton, "Initiation of Sexual Activity"; Frank F. Furstenberg, "As the Pendulum Swings: Teenage Childbearing and Social Concern," *Family Relations* 40 (1991): 127–38; Velma McBride Murry, "Incidence of First Pregnancy among Black Adolescent Females over Three Decades," *Youth and Society* 23, no. 4 (1992): 478–506; Wallace and Bachman, "Explaining Racial/Ethnic Differences."

19. Feldman, *Culture.*

20. Jones, *Teenage Pregnancy*; Zelnik et al., *Sex and Pregnancy.*

21. Forste and Heaton, "Initiation of Sexual Activity."

22. Dryfoos, *Adolescents at Risk.*

23. Jones, *Teenage Pregnancy*; Ladner, *Tomorrow's Tomorrow*; Frank Furstenberg, Richard Lincoln, and F. Menken, eds., *Teenage Sexuality, Pregnancy and Childbearing* (Philadelphia: University of Philadelphia Press, 1981).

24. Rosenheim and Testa, eds., *Early Parenthood.*

25. Murry, "First Pregnancy."

26. Lowenstein and Furstenberg, "Is Teenage Sexual Behavior Rational?"

27. Koyle, "Comparison of Sexual Behaviors"; Gordon, "Adolescent Sexuality"; Vivian T. Shayne and Barbara J. Kaplan, "AIDS Education for Adolescents," *Youth and Society* 20, no. 2 (1988): 180–208; Wallace, "Racial/Ethnic Differences."

28. Edelman and Ladner, *Adolescence*; Luker, *Dubious Conceptions*.

29. Moore and Rosenthal, *Sexuality*; Rosenheim and Testa, eds., *Early Parenthood*.

30. Luker, *Dubious Conceptions*.

31. Janie Victoria Ward, "Raising Resisters: The Role of Truth-Telling in the Psychological Development of African American Girls," in *Urban Girls*, Leadbeater and Way, eds. 85–99.

32. This sense of responsibility does not include considering masturbation as a viable sexual option. None of the participants were willing to admit ever even thinking of, as one put it, "doing something so totally nasty."

33. Within social psychology, theorists (see John De Lamater and Patricia MacCorqodale, *Premarital Sexuality: Attitudes, Relationships, Behavior* [Madison: University of Wisconsin Press, 1979]; Kaplan et al., "Sociological Study") define individuals who believe that they have control over their social environment and thus control of their lives as having high self-efficacy or an internal locus of control. Individuals from socially and economically secure families rate higher levels of self-efficacy and locus of control than individuals from less secure situations. However, teenagers from less economically stable backgrounds regularly score high on measures of self-esteem or self-concept (Cairns and Cairns, *Lifelines*).

34. Karl E. Bauman and J. Richard Udry, "Subjective Expected Utility and Adolescent Sexual Behavior," *Adolescence* 16, no. 63 (1981): 527–35; Koyle et al., "Comparison of Sexual Behaviors."

35. Fox, "The Family's Role."

36. Nathanson, *Dangerous Passage*.

37. In a survey of sexually active black men and women, *Essence* magazine (September 1994) reported that many adults, both male and female, find oral sex aberrant sexual behavior. Even so, both men and women reported wanting more oral sex in their relationships.

38. Benjamin Bowser, Mindy Thompson Fullilove, and Robert E. Fullilove, "African American Youth and High Risk Behavior: The Social Context and Barriers to Prevention," *Youth and Society* 22, no. 1 (1990): 54–66; Murry, "Incident of First Pregnancy"; Wallace and Bachman, "Racial/Ethnic Differences"; Washington, "A Cultural and Historical Perspective."

39. Anderson, *Streetwise*; William Julius Wilson, *The Truly Disadvantaged* (Chicago: University of Chicago Press, 1987).

40. Forste and Heaton, "Initiation of Sexual Activity"; Furstenberg, "As the Pendulum Swings"; Murry "Incidence of First Pregnancy"; Wallace, "Explaining Racial/Ethnic Differences."

41. It is important to note that teenagers with children are more likely to be poor than teenagers without children, and that birth rates are highest among

poor teens (Geronimus, "Social Disadvantage"; Zelnik et al., *Sex and Pregnancy*; Nathanson, *Dangerous Passage*). The social isolation and alienation from institutions that these young women experienced may explain some of their distrust of the health care system.

42. Caroline Wolf Harlow, *Female Victims of Violent Crime* (Washington, D.C.: U.S. Department of Justice, 1991).

43. See my essay "In the Name of Love and Survival" for a description of typologies used by young women to define different kinds of sexual violence, ranging from sex play to coercion, rape, and violence. They often defined sexual violence at the hands of an intimate partner as sex play.

44. Anderson, *Streetwise*; Feldman, *Culture and AIDS*; Wilson, *The Truly Disadvantaged*.

45. Arlie Hochschild, *The Second Shift: Work, Parenting, and the Revolution at Home* (New York: Viking, 1989).

46. This perception is illustrated in Evelyn and Rhonda's comments in the previous section. See also Collins, *Black Feminist Thought*, and Rosalind Petchesky, "Reproductive Freedom: Beyond a Woman's Right to Choose," *Signs* 5 (1980): 661–85.

47. Patricia Spallone, *Beyond Conception: The New Politics of Reproduction* (Granby, Mass.: Bergin and Garvey, 1989), 17.

48. Susan Bram, "The Effects of Childbearing on Women's Mental Health: A Critical Review of the Literature," in *Genes and Gender IV: The Second X and Women's Health*, ed. Myra Fooden, Susan Gordon, and Betty Highley (New York: Gordian, 1983); Levine, "AIDS and Changing Concepts."

49. Geronimus, "Social Disadvantage"; Lowenstein and Furstenberg, "Is Teenage Sexual Behavior Rational?"; Thompson, *Going All the Way*.

50. Paul Crosbie and Dianne Bitte, "A Test of Luker's Theory of Contraceptive Risk–Taking," *Studies in Family Planning* 13, no. 3 (1989): 205–27.

51. Feldman, *Culture and AIDS*.

Chapter 6

1. Arthur A. Campbell and Wendy Baldwin, "The Response of American Women to the Threat of AIDS and Other STDs," *Journal on AIDS* 4 (1990): 1133–40; Nathanson, *Dangerous Passage*.

2. Fan et al., *AIDS*, 184.

3. Lowenstein and Furstenberg, "Is Teenage Sexual Behavior Rational?"; William D. Mosher and James W. McNally, "Contraceptive Use at First Premarital Intercourse: United States, 1965–1988," *Family Planning Perspectives* 23, no. 3 (1991): 108–16; Freya L. Sonenstein, Joseph Pleck, and Leighton C. Ku, "Sexual Activity, Condom Use and AIDS Awareness among Adolescent Males," *Family Planning Perspectives* 21, no. 4 (1989): 152–58.

4. Mosher and McNally, "Contraceptive Use."

5. Zelnik et al., *Sex and Pregnancy*.

6. Since this study was conducted before the advent of AIDS, Zelnik et al.

defined condom use as a nonmedical barrier method. I would argue that any contraceptive method that minimizes or eradicates the risk of HIV infection is in fact a medical contraceptive. Defining the input of a medical professional for contraception as a medical intervention dilutes the amount of power a person has over his or her sexuality by minimizing the importance of self-determination in preventive behavior.

7. I am qualifying this claim because on a few occasions young women described instances when they borrowed birth control pills from a friend. Perhaps they had no physician or did not want to discuss their sexual activity with their doctor. Their understanding of the purpose of the pill was unclear. They believed that its effectiveness was situational, not cumulative; just as an individual takes a pill for a headache, a woman takes a pill whenever she plans on having sex in order to prevent pregnancy. This approach is very different from taking one pill every single day. By maintaining this perspective, the young woman with the prescription as well as any of her "pill borrowers" are at an even greater risk of pregnancy.

8. Jones et al., *Teenage Pregnancy*.

9. Jones et al., *Teenage Pregnancy*, 51.

10. Lowenstein and Furstenberg, "Is Teenage Sexual Behavior Rational?"

11. Mosher and McNally, "Contraceptive Use," 115.

12. Shayne and Kaplan, "AIDS Education."

13. Elicia Herz and Janet S. Reis, "Family Life Education for Young Inner-City Teens: Identifying Needs," *Journal of Youth and Adolescence* 16, no. 4 (1987): 361–76.

14. Collins, *Black Feminist Thought*; K. Sue Jewell, *From Mammy to Miss America and Beyond: Cultural Images and the Shaping of U.S. Social Policy* (New York: Routledge, 1993).

15. Sonenstein et al., "Sexual Activity."

16. Centers for Disease Control, *Facts about Adolescents and AIDS* (Atlanta: CDC Division of HIV/AIDS, December 1995).

17. Behavior change is defined as stopping one of the following behaviors: intercourse, other sexual relations, frequent sexual activity, multiple sexual partners, casual sex, bisexual sexual contacts, or sex with intravenous drug users (*NCHS Advance Data*, December 1993, #239).

18. Mosher and McNally, "Contraceptive Use."

19. Thomas Andre and Lynda Bormann, "Knowledge of Acquired Immune Deficiency Syndrome and Sexual Responsibility among High School Students," *Youth and Society* 22, no. 3 (1991): 339–61; Leslie R. Jaffe, Mavis Seehaus, Claudia Wagner, and Bonnie Leadbeater, "Anal Intercourse and Knowledge of Acquired Immune Deficiency Syndrome among Minority-Group Female Adolescents," *Journal of Pediatrics* 112, no. 6 (1988): 1005–7; Lowenstein and Furstenberg, "Is Teenage Sexual Behavior Rational?"

20. Mosher and McNally, "Contraceptive Use"; Sonenstein et al., "Sexual Activity."

21. Gordon and Gilgun, "Adolescent Sexuality."

22. Campbell, "The Response"; Sonenstein et al., "Sexual Activity."

23. Lisa G. Aspinwall, Margaret Kemeny, Shelley Taylor, Stephen Schneider, and Janice Dudley, "Psychosocial Predictors of Gay Men's AIDS Risk Reduction Behavior," *Health Psychology* 10, no. 6 (1991): 432–44; Joseph Catania, Susan M. Kegeles, and Thomas Coates, "Towards an Understanding of Risk Behavior: An AIDS Risk Reduction Model," *Health Education Quarterly* 17, no. 1 (1990): 53–72.

24. Campbell and Baldwin, "The Response," 1137.

25. De La Cancela, "Minority AIDS Prevention"; Dryfoos, *Adolescents at Risk*.

26. This recent high school graduate has sex with three men on a weekly basis and uses no contraception. Her interest in abstaining from further sex is becoming more popular among sexually active women of all ages. There is a new wave of "born again" and "rededicated" virgins. One young woman even called this decision "reinvirgination."

27. Also see Deena's description of sex at parties in chapter 5.

28. Willard Cates, "Teenagers and Risk Taking: The Best of Times and the Worst of Times," *Journal of Adolescent Health* 12 (1991): 84–94; Edelgard Wulfert and Choi K. Wan, "Safer Sex Intentions and Condom Use, Viewed from a Health Belief, Reasoned Action and Social Cognitive Perspective," *Journal of Sex Research* 32, no. 4 (1995): 299–311.

29. Joan A. Jurich, Rebecca A. Adams, and John E. Schulenberg, "Factors Related to Behavior Change in Response to AIDS," *Family Relations* 41 (1992): 97–103.

30. Andre and Bormann, "Knowledge"; Lowenstein and Furstenberg, "Is Teenage Sexual Behavior Rational?"

31. G. Stephen Bowen, Sevgi O. Aral, Lawrence S. Magder, Deborah S. Reed, Cathy Dratmen, and Shari C. Wasser, "Risk Behaviors for HIV Infection in Clients of Pennsylvania Family Planning Clinics," *Family Planning Perspectives* 22 (1990): 62–64; Dryfoos, *Adolescents at Risk*; Lowenstein and Furstenberg, "Is Teenage Sexual Behavior Rational?"; Zelnik et al., *Sex and Pregnancy*.

32. Dooley Worth, "Minority Women and AIDS: Culture, Race, and Gender," in *Culture and AIDS*, ed. Douglas Feldman (New York: Praeger, 1990), 111–35.

33. Vickie M. Mays and Susan C. Cochran, "Issues in the Perception of AIDS Risk and Risk Reduction Activities by Black and Hispanic/Latina Women," *American Psychologist* 43 (1988): 949–57.

34. Worth, "Minority Women and AIDS," 111.

35. Herz and Reis, "Family Life Education."

36. Wendy Chavkin, "Women, AIDS and Reproductive Rights: Preventing AIDS, Targeting Women," *Health Pac Bulletin* (1990): 19–23; Shayne, "AIDS Education."

37. Sonenstein et al., "Sexual Activity."

38. Bowser et al., "African American Youth"; Chavkin, "Women, AIDS."

39. De La Cancela, "Minority AIDS Prevention"; Dryfoos, *Adolescents at Risk*; Furstenberg, "As the Pendulum Swings."

40. Jaffe, "Anal Intercourse," 1007.

41. This should not be confused with the conservative argument that one's life is solely determined by hard work. Such an argument denies the way institutions can constrain opportunity in spite of an individual's commitment and positive outlook. What I am arguing is that perceptions influence motivation but that the reality of one's life, the presence of institutional supports to facilitate one's future, will ultimately affect behavior.

42. Klein, "Adolescence, Youth"; Nathanson, *Dangerous Passage*.

43. Campbell and Baldwin, "The Response."

Chapter 7

1. Office of National AIDS Policy, *Youth and HIV/AIDS: An American Agenda—A Report to the President* (Washington, D.C.: National AIDS Fund, 1986), 2–3.

2. John E. Anderson, Laura Kann, Deborah Holtzman, Susan Arday, Ben Truman, and Lloyd Kolbe, "Knowledge of Acquired Immune Deficiency Syndrome and Sexual Responsibility Among High School Students," *Youth and Society* 22, no. 3 (1991): 339–61.

3. Andre and Bormann, "Knowledge"; Rosemary A. Jadack, Janet S. Hyde, and Mary Keller, "Gender and Knowledge about HIV, Risky Sexual Behavior and Safer Sex Practices," *Research in Nursing Health* 18, no. 4 (1995): 313–24.

4. Richie, "AIDS."

5. National Institutes of Health, "HIV/AIDS-Related Research Program at the National Institutes of Health," http://www.os.dhhs.gov/ (October 4, 1996).

6. One black, middle-class woman described an encounter with a private physician. The gynecologist, a white male, was supposed to complete her annual exam. His first few questions, presumably an attempt to generate her medical and sexual history, offended her. He asked her to describe in detail the sexual contacts she had in the past few years. He asked her whether she had multiple orgasms and told her that she probably had AIDS because of her past. This woman was active in the health care community and knew that his diagnosis was inappropriate. In relaying this story to me, she noted that at least she could find another physician. She wondered about less well-informed women who might either remain with an ineffective doctor or be frightened away and avoid further care. From her contact with low-income women in New Haven, she concluded that her experience was very common.

7. Laraine Winter and Lynne Cooper Brekenmaker, "Tailoring Family Planning Services to the Special Needs of Adolescents," *Family Planning Perspectives* 23, no. 1 (1991): 24–30.

8. Mays and Cochran, "Issues in the Perception"; Earl E. Schelp, Edwin DuBose, and Ronald Sunderland, "AIDS and the Church: A Status Report," *Christian Century* 107, no. 35 (1990): 1135–37.

9. Centers for Disease Control, "Facts."

10. Bayer, "AIDS and the Future"; Chavkin, "Women, AIDS"; T. Richard Sullivan, "The Challenge of HIV Prevention among High–Risk Adolescents," *Health and Social Work* 21, no. 1 (1996): 58–65.

11. Karen J. Pittman, "Reading and Writing as Risk Reduction: The School's Role in Preventing Teenage Pregnancies," in *Teenage Pregnancy*, ed. Elise F. Jones, et al.

12. Rebecca Adams, Fred P. Piercy, Joan J. Jurich, and Robert A. Lewis, "Components of a Model Adolescent AIDS/Drug Abuse Prevention Program: A Delphi Study," *Family Relations* 41 (1992): 314.

13. Fine, "Sexuality, Schooling"; Nathanson, *Dangerous Passage*; Schinke et al., "African-American."

14. "Studies Find School Condom Programs Don't Promote Sex," *AIDS Policy Law* 10, no. 15 (August 1995): 8.

15. "Court Upholds 'Hot and Sexy' AIDS Education Campaign," *AIDS Policy Law* 10, no. 21 (December 1995): 1, 11.

16. J. L. Matzen, "Assessment of Human Immunodeficiency Virus/Acquired Immunodeficiency Syndrome Audiovisual Activities by Black and Hispanic/Latina Women," *Journal of Pediatric Nursing* 10, no. 2 (1995): 114–20; Roberta Weiner, *AIDS: Impact on the Schools* (Arlington, Va.: Education Research Group, 1986).

17. She later explained that AIDS was contracted from sex and that people with AIDS looked sick. She was unable to make the distinction between a healthy-looking person with HIV or AIDS and the images of late-stage AIDS patients she had seen in photos. In her view, all HIV-infected people looked like "really gross, sick . . . people."

18. Kathleen Ford and Anne Norris, "Urban African-American and Hispanic Adolescents and Young Adults: Who Do They Talk to about AIDS and Condoms? What Are They Learning?" *AIDS Education and Prevention* 3, no. 3 (1991): 197–206.

19. See Dominique Moyse-Steinberg, "A Model for Adolescent Pregnancy Prevention through the Use of Small Groups," *Social Work with Groups* 13, no. 2 (1990): 57–68, for an example of the benefits of small peer groups in prevention initiatives.

20. Stephen R. Jorgensen, "Sex Education and the Reduction of Adolescent Pregnancies: Prospects for the 1980s," *Journal of Early Adolescence* 1, no. 1 (1981): 48–49.

21. DiClemente, "Predictors"; Jeffrey A. Kelly, Janet St. Lawrence, Yolanda E. Diaz, L. Yvonne Stevenson, Allan C. Hauth, Ted L. Brasfield, Seth C. Kalichman, Joseph E. Smith, and Michael E. Andrews, "HIV Risk Behavior Reduction Following Interviews with Key Opinion Leaders of the Population: An Experimental Analysis," *American Journal of Public Health* 81, no. 2 (1991): 168–71; Sol Levine and James Sorenson, "Social and Cultural Factors in Health Promotion," in *Behavioral Health: A Handbook of Health Enhancement and Disease Prevention*, ed. J. D. Matarazzo, S. M. Weiss, J. A. Herd, N. E. Miller (New York: Wiley, 1984).

22. Melinda Tuhus, "Our Youth at Risk: Children, Sex and Death in the

Age of AIDS," *New Times Connecticut* (November 28/December 5, 1991): 8–12, 14.

23. These clinics can be found in thirty-two states (Douglas E. Kirby, Cynthia Waszak, and Julie Ziegler, "Six School-Based Clinics: Their Reproductive Health Services and Impact on Sexual Behavior," *Family Planning Perspectives* 23, no. 1 [1991]: 6–16).

24. See Jonathan Mann and Daniel Tarantola, eds., *AIDS in the World II: Global Dimensions, Social Roots, and Responses* (New York: Oxford University Press, 1996); Heather G. Miller, Charles F. Turner, and Lincoln E. Moses, eds., *AIDS: The Second Decade* (Washington, D.C.: National Academy Press, 1990).

25. Musick, *Young, Poor*, 131.

26. Winter and Brekenmaker, "Tailoring Family Planning."

27. Mays and Cochran, "Issues in Perception."

28. Bayer, "AIDS and the Future."

29. De La Cancela, "Minority AIDS Prevention"; Weeks et al., AIDS Prevention."

30. Jill G. Joseph, Carol Ann Emmons, Ronald Kessler, Camille B. Wortman, Keith O'Brien, William T. Hocker, and Catherine Schaefer, "Coping with the Threat of AIDS: An Approach to Psychosocial Assessment," *American Psychologist* 39 (1984): 11–21; Moyse–Steinberg, "A Model."

31. Floyd Hayes, in political science and African-American studies at Purdue University, is currently studying a phenomenon he calls "urban cynicism." Youth of color who have become politically and emotionally alienated from social institutions begin to disengage from "traditional" behavior because they realize that they are systematically excluded from opportunities. This attitude is different from fatalism, which implies not only that youth are disconnected from society but that they actively engage in destructive behaviors because they have no sense of a future. In Hayes's conceptualization, youth are agents in their own future. They reject the mainstream in search of innovative alternatives.

32. De La Cancela, "Minority AIDS Prevention," 146.

33. Forste and Heaton, "Initiation."

34. Marvin Eisen, Gail L. Zellman, and Alfred L. McAlister, "Evaluating the Impact of a Theory–Based Sexuality and Contraceptive Education Program," *Family Planning Perspectives* 22, no. 6 (1990): 261–71.

35. Laurie Schwab Zabin and Marilyn B. Hirsch, *Evaluation of Pregnancy Prevention Programs in the School Context* (Lexington, Mass: Lexington Books, 1988).

36. Amaro," Love"; Ralph J. DiClemente and G. M. Wingood, "A Randomized Controlled Trial of an HIV Sexual Risk–Reduction Intervention for Young African-American Women," *Journal of the American Medical Association* 274, no. 16 (1995): 1271–76.

37. Diane Scott-Jones, "Adolescent Childbearing: Risk and Resilience," *Education and Urban Society* 24, no. 1 (1991): 53–64; Shayne and Kaplan, "AIDS Education."

38. "Standing Up for Yourself, Good Communication Will Help You Get

Your Partner to Use a Condom," *AIDS Alert* 10, no. 12 (December 1995): Suppl. 1–2; Vered Slonim–Nevo, Martha N. Ozawa, and Wendy F. Auslander, "Knowledge, Attitudes and Behavior Related to AIDS among Youth in Residential Centers: Results from an Explanatory Study," *Journal of Adolescence* 14 (1991): 17–33.

39. Schinke et al., "African-American."

40. Allen et al., "School Based Prevention"; Forste and Heaton, "Initiation of Sexual Activity"; Mays and Cochran, "Issues."

41. Cates, "Teenagers and Risk Taking."

42. Shayne and Kaplan, "AIDS Education."

43. Adams et al., "Components of a Model"; Anderson, "HIV/AIDS Knowledge."

44. Eisen et al., "Evaluating the Impact"; Kirby, "Six School-Based Clinics"; Winter and Brekenmaker, "Tailoring Family Planning."

45. Sevgi O. Aral, Lawrence S. Magder, and G. Stephen Bowen, "HIV Risk Behavior Screening: Concordance between Assessments through Interviews and Questionnaires," *Fifth Conference on AIDS Abstracts* (Ottowa, Canada: International Development Research Centre, 1989); DiClemente, "Predictors"; Jurich, "Factors Related."

46. Thomas J. Coates, "Strategies for Modifying Sexual Behavior for Primary and Secondary Prevention of HIV Disease," *Journal of Counseling and Clinical Psychology* 58, no. 1 (1990): 66.

47. Coates, "Strategies," 66.

48. Shayne and Kaplan, "AIDS Education," 202.

49. Schinke et al., "African-American."

50. De La Cancela, "Minority AIDS Prevention."

51. Ford and Norris, "Urban African-American."

52. Joyce Ladner, "Black Teenage Pregnancy: A Challenge for Educators," *Journal of Negro Education* 56, no. 1 (1987): 58.

53. Steven E. Keller, Jacqueline Bertlett, Steven J. Schleifer, Robert L. Johnson, Elizabeth Pinner, and Beverly Delaney, "HIV Relevant Sexual Behavior among a Healthy Inner-City Heterosexual Adolescent Population in an Endemic Area of HIV," *Journal of Adolescent Health* 12 (1991): 44–48.

54. Marte and Anastos, "Women—Part II," 15.

Chapter 8

1. Richie, "AIDS."

2. Marte and Anastos, "Women—Part I."

3. Robert J. Taylor, "African-American Inner City Youth and Subculture," in *Teenage Pregnancy*," ed. Jones and Battle, 16.

4. Anderson, *Streetwise*; Dash, *When Children*; Jencks and Peterson, *The Urban Underclass*; Ladner, *Tomorrow's Tomorrow*; Stack, *All Our Kin*; Wilson, *The Truly Disadvantaged*.

5. *Black Power* (New York: Vintage Books, 1992), 159–60.

6. Roderick Wallace and Deborah Wallace, "Contagious Urban Decay and the Collapse of Public Health," *Health/PAC Bulletin* (Summer 1991): 13–18. See also Washington, "A Cultural and Historical Perspective."

7. Adalberto Aguirre and Jonathan H. Turner, *American Ethnicity* (New York: McGraw-Hill, 1995); Paul Peterson, ed., *The New Urban Reality* (Washington, D.C.: Brookings, 1985), 225–52; Wilson, *The Truly Disadvantaged*.

8. Edelman and Ladner, *Adolescence and Poverty*, 114.

9. M. Witwer, "Pregnancy Risk Lessened for Teenagers with High Educational Aspirations," *Family Planning Perspectives* 25, no. 4 (1993): 189–90.

10. Wallace and Bachman, "Explaining Racial/Ethnic Differences."

11. Harris, *Teen Pregnancy*.

12. Jacquelyn H. Flaskerud and Adeline M. Nyamathi, "Black and Latina Women's AIDS Related Knowledge, Attitudes, and Practices," *Research in Nursing and Health* 12 (1989): 339–46.

References

Abdul-Salaam, Mustapha. *About the New Haven Family Alliance.* New Haven, Conn.: New Haven Family Alliance, 1991.

Abraham, Laurie. "Pregnant Women Face AIDS Dilemma." *American Medical News* 22 (July 1988): 3, 34–35.

Adams, Rebecca A., Fred P. Piercy, Joan A. Jurich, and Robert A. Lewis. "Components of a Model Adolescent AIDS/Drug Abuse Prevention Program: A Delphi Study." *Family Relations* 41 (1992): 312–17.

Adib, Maurice, Jill G. Joseph, David G. Ostrow, Margalit Tal, and Stanley A. Schwartz. "Relapse in Sexual Behavior among Homosexual Men: A Two Year Follow Up from the Chicago MACS/CCS." *AIDS* 5 (1991): 757–60.

Aguirre, Adalberto, and Jonathan H. Turner. *American Ethnicity.* New York: McGraw-Hill, 1995.

AIDS Alert. "Community Interventions Double Condom Use among African-Americans." 10, no. 12 (1995): 145–47.

———. "NICHD Researches Women's Attitudes, Behavior." 11, no. 3 (1996): 31.

———. "Standing Up for Yourself, Good Communication Will Help You Get Your Partner to Use a Condom." 10, no. 12 (1995): Suppl. 1–2.

AIDS Policy Law. "Studies Find School Condom Programs Don't Promote Sex." 10, no. 15 (1995): 8.

———. "Court Upholds 'Hot and Sexy' AIDS Education Campaign." 10, no. 21 (1995): 1, 11.

Allen, Joseph P., Susan Philliber, and Nancy Hoggson. "School Based Prevention of Teen-Age Pregnancy and School Dropout: Process Evaluation of National Replication of Teen Outreach Programs." *American Journal of Community Psychology* 18, no. 4 (1990): 505–24.

Alonso, Ana Maria, and Maria Teresa Koreck. "Silences: 'Hispanics,' AIDS, and Sexual Practices." *Differences* 2 (1989): 101–24.

Amaro, Hortensia. "Love, Sex, and Power: Considering Women's Realities in HIV Prevention." *American Psychologist* 50, no. 6 (1995): 437–47.

Anderson, Elaine A. "AIDS Public Policy: Implications for Families." *New England Journal of Public Policy* 4 (1988): 411–27.

Anderson, Elijah. *Streetwise: Race, Class and Change in an Urban City.* Chicago: University of Chicago, 1990.

Anderson, John E., Laura Kann, Deborah Holtzman, Susan Arday, Ben Truman, and Lloyd Kolbe. "HIV/AIDS Knowledge and Behavior Among High School Students." *Family Planning Perspectives* 22, no. 6 (November/December 1990): 252–55.

Andre, Thomas, and Lynda Bormann. "Knowledge of Acquired Immune Deficiency Syndrome and Sexual Responsibility among High School Students." *Youth and Society* 22, no. 3 (1991): 339–61.

Angell, Marcia. "A Dual Approach to the AIDS Epidemic." *The New England Journal of Medicine* 324, no. 21 (1991): 1498–500.

Annas, George. "Protecting the Liberty of Pregnant Patients." *New England Journal of Medicine* 316 (1987): 121–14.

Ansuini, Catherine G., Robert Woite, and Julianna Fiddler Woite. "The Source, Accuracy, and Impact of Initial Sexuality Information on Lifetime Wellness." *Adolescence* 31, no. 122 (1996): 238–89.

Aral, Sevgi O., Lawrence S. Magder, and G. Stephen Bowen. "HIV Risk Behavior Screening: Concordance between Assessments through Interviews and Questionnaires." *Fifth Conference on AIDS Abstracts.* Ottawa, Canada: International Development Research Center, 1989.

Arditi, Rita, Renata Duelli Klein, and Shelley Minden. *Test Tube Women: What Future for Motherhood?* London: Pandora, 1984.

Aronson, Elliot, Carrie Fried, and Jeff Stone. "Overcoming Denial and Increasing the Intention to Use Condoms through Induction of Hypocrisy." *American Journal of Public Health* 81, no. 12 (1991): 1636–38.

Aspinwall, Lisa G., Margaret Kemeny, Shelley Taylor, Stephen Schneider, and Janice Dudley. "Psychosocial Predictors of Gay Men's AIDS Risk Reduction Behavior." *Health Psychology* 10, no. 6 (1991): 432–44.

Avery, Byllye. "Black Woman's Health: A Conspiracy of Silence." *Sojourner* 14 (1989): 15.

Bachu, Amara. *Fertility of American Women.* Washington, D.C: U.S. Bureau of the Census, 1993.

Bandura, Albert. *Social Learning Theory.* Upper Saddle River, N.J.: Prentice Hall, 1977.

Barnett, Jawanda K., Dennis R. Papini, and Edward Gbur. "Familial Correlates of Sexually Active Pregnant and Nonpregnant Adolescents." *Adolescence* 26, no. 102 (1991): 457–72.

Battle, Stanley F. "Teenage Pregnancy and Out of Wedlock Births." In *Teenage Pregnancy: Developmental Strategies for Change in the Twenty First Century,* ed. Dionne J. Jones and Stanley F. Battle. New Brunswick, N.J.: Transaction, 1990.

Bauman, Karl E., and J. Richard Udry. "Subjective Expected Utility and Adolescent Sexual Behavior." *Adolescence* 16, no. 63 (1981): 527–35.

Bayer, Ronald. "Public Health Policy and the AIDS Epidemic–An End to AIDS Exceptionalism?" *New England Journal of Medicine* 324, no. 21 (1991): 1500–4.

———. "AIDS and the Future of Reproductive Freedom." *Milbank Quarterly* 68 Suppl., no. 2 (1990): 179–204.

———. "The Suitability of HIV-Positive Individuals for Marriage and Pregnancy." *Journal of the American Medical Association* 261 (1989): 993.

Beck, Kenneth, and Adrian K. Lund. "The Effects of Health Threat Seriousness and Personal Efficacy upon Intentions and Behavior." *Journal of Applied Social Psychology* 11 (1981): 401–15.

Becker, Marshall H. "Psychosocial Aspects of Health Related Behavior." In *Handbook of Medical Sociology*, 3d ed., ed. H. Freeman, S. Levine, and L. Reeder. Upper Saddle River, N.J.: Prentice Hall, 1990.

———. "The Tyranny of Health Promotion." *Public Health Reviews* 14 (1986): 15–25.

Becker, Marshall H., and Jill G. Joseph. "AIDS and Behavior Change to Reduce Risk: A Review." *American Journal of Public Health* 78, no. 4 (1988): 394–410.

Bennett, Neil G., David E. Bloom, and Cynthia K. Miller. "The Influence of Nonmarital Childbearing on the Formation of First Marriages." *Demography* 32, no. 1 (1995): 47–62.

Blackwell, James E. *The Black Community: Diversity and Unity*. New York: Harper & Row, 1985.

Blattner, William A. "HIV Epidemiology: Past, Present and Future." *The FASEB Journal* 5 (1991): 2340–48.

Blum, Henrik L. "Social Perspective on Risk Reduction." In *Promoting Health through Risk Reduction*, ed. M. Faber and A. Reinhardt. New York: Macmillan, 1982.

Bowen, G. Stephen, Sevgi O. Aral, Lawrence S. Magder, Deborah S. Reed, Cathy Dratmen, and Shari C. Wasser. "Risk Behaviors for HIV Infection in Clients of Pennsylvania Family Planning Clinics." *Family Planning Perspectives* 22 (1990): 62–64.

Bowser, Benjamin, Mindy Thompson Fullilove, and Robert E. Fullilove. "African-American Youth and High Risk Behavior: The Social Context and Barriers to Prevention." *Youth and Society* 22, no. 1 (1990): 54–66.

Bram, Susan. "The Effects of Childbearing on Women's Mental Health: A Critical Review of the Literature." In *Genes and Gender IV: The Second X and Women's Health*, ed. Myra Fooden, Susan Gordon, and Betty Hughley. New York: Gordian, 1983.

Brooks-Gunn, Jeanne, and Frank F. Furstenberg. "Adolescent Sexual Behavior." *American Psychologist* 44, no. 2 (1989): 249–57.

Brooks-Gunn, Jeanne, and Frank F. Furstenberg, Jr. "Coming of Age in the Era of AIDS: Puberty, Sexuality and Contraception." *Milbank Quarterly* 68 Suppl. (1990): 59–84.

Brown, Lawrence S., and Beny J. Primm. "Intravenous Drug Abuse and AIDS in Minorities." *AIDS and Public Policy Journal* 3 (1988): 5–15.

Brown, Shirley Vining. "Premarital Sexual Permissiveness among Black Adolescent Females." *Social Psychology Quarterly* 48, no. 4 (1985): 381–87.

Browne, Margaret. "Teenage Pregnancy and the Sexist Image." *Genes and Gender* 3 (1980): 150–59.

Brownell, Kelly D., G. Alan Markatt, Edward Lichenstein, and Terence Wilson. "Understanding and Preventing Relapse." *American Psychologist* 41, no. 7 (1986): 765–82.

Burawoy, Michael. *Ethnography Unbound: Power and Resistance in the Modern Metropolis*. Berkeley: University of California Press, 1991.

Butts, June Dobbs. "Adolescent Sexuality and Teenage Pregnancy from a Black Perspective." In *Teenage Pregnancy in a Family Context*, ed. Theodora Ooms. Philadelphia: Temple University Press, 1981.

Cairns, Robert B., and Beverly D. Cairns. *Lifelines and Risk: Pathways of Youth in Our Time*. Cambridge: Cambridge University Press, 1994.

Campbell, Arthur A., and Wendy Baldwin. "The Response of American Women to the Threat of AIDS and Other STDs." *Journal on AIDS* 4 (1990): 1133–40.

Cartoof, Virginia G. *Evaluation of the Hill Health Center's Young Parents' Outreach Program, 1983–1990*. Dorchester, Mass.: Cartoof Consulting, 1991.

Cassens, Brett J. "Social Consequences of the Acquired Immunodeficiency Syndrome—United States." *Annals of Internal Medicine* 103 (1985): 768–71.

Catania, Joseph A., Valerie Stone, Diane Binson, and M. Margaret Dolcini. "Changes in Condom Use among Heterosexuals in Wave 3 of the AMEN Study." *The Journal of Sex Research* 32, no. 3 (1995): 193–200.

Catania, Joseph A., Susan M. Kegeles, and Thomas J. Coates. "Towards an Understanding of Risk Behavior: An AIDS Risk Reduction Model (ARRM)." *Health Education Quarterly* 17, no. 1 (1990): 53–72.

Cates, Willard. "Teenagers and Risk Taking: The Best of Times and the Worst of Times." *Journal of Adolescent Health* 12 (1991): 84–94.

Center for Population Options. "Adolescent Sexuality, Pregnancy and Parenthood." Washington, D.C.: CPO, May 1990a.

———. "Adolescents and Abortion." Washington, D.C.: CPO, May 1990b.

Centers for Disease Control (CDC). *Behavioral and Prevention Research Branch: Summary of MMWR Articles 1992–1993*. Atlanta: CDC Division of HIV/AIDS, 1993.

———. "Facts about Adolescents and AIDS." Atlanta: CDC Division of HIV/AIDS, December 1995.

———. "Guidelines for Health Education and Risk Reduction Activities." http://wonder.cdc.gov/rchtml/convert/std/RHER3708.pcw.html, 1995.

———. *HIV/AIDS Surveillance*. hhtp://www.cdc.gov, March 1998.

———. *HIV/AIDS Surveillance Year End Edition*. Atlanta: CDC Division of HIV/AIDS, 1992.

Chavkin, Wendy. "Women, AIDS and Reproductive Rights: Preventing AIDS, Targeting Women." *Health/Pac Bulletin* Spring (1990): 19–23.

Checko, Patricia J., Julia Wang Miller, and Clare Averbach. "The Epidemiology of AIDS in Connecticut." *Connecticut Medicine* 55, no. 1 (1991): 3–8.

Chirimuuta, Rosalind J. Harrison, and Richard C. Chirimuuta. "AIDS from Africa: A Case of Racism vs. Science?" In *AIDS in Africa and the Caribbean*, ed. George C. Bond, John Kreniske, Ida Susser, and Joan Vincent. Boulder, Colo.: Westview, 1997.

Chodorow, Nancy. *The Reproduction of Mothering*. Berkeley: University of California Press, 1978.

Christensen, Harold T., and Leanor B. Johnson. "Premarital Coitus and the

Southern Black: A Comparative View." *Journal of Marriage and the Family* 40 (1978): 721–32.

Clark, Susan, Laurie Sabin, and Janet Hardy. "Sex Contraception and Parenthood: Experiences and Attitudes among Urban Black Young Men." *Family Planning Perspectives* 16 (1984): 77–82.

Coates, Thomas J. "Strategies for Modifying Sexual Behavior for Primary and Secondary Prevention of HIV Disease." *Journal of Consulting and Clinical Psychology* 58, no. 1 (1990): 57–69.

Coates, Thomas J., Lydia Temoshok, and Jeffrey Mandel. "Psychosocial Research is Essential to Understanding and Treating AIDS." *American Psychologist* 39, no. 11 (1984): 1309–14.

Cochran, Susan D., Vickie M. Mays, and V. Roberts. "Ethnic Minorities and AIDS." In *Nursing Care of the Patient with AIDS/ARC*, ed. A. Lewis. Rockville, Md.: Aspen, 1988.

Cohen, Felissa, and Jerry Durham. *Women, Children and HIV/AIDS.* New York: Springer, 1993.

Cohen, Sheldon, and S. Leonard Syme. *Social Support and Health.* New York: Academic Press, 1985.

Cohen, Stuart. "Intentional Teenage Pregnancies." *Journal of School Health* 53, no. 3 (1983): 210–11.

Collins, Patricia Hill. *Black Feminist Thought.* Boston: Unwin Hyman, 1990.

Connecticut Department of Public Health. *AIDS in Connecticut: Annual Surveillance Report, December 31, 1993.* Hartford: Department of Public Health, AIDS Epidemiology Program, 1994.

——. *AIDS in Connecticut: Annual Surveillance Report, December 31, 1996.* Hartford: Department of Public Health, AIDS Epidemiology Program, 1997.

Connecticut Economic Information System (CEIS). http://www.state.ct.us/ecd/research/ceis/, March 1998.

Corea, Gena. *The Mother Machine.* New York: Harper & Row, 1985.

Crane, Jonathan. "Effects of Neighborhoods on Dropping Out of School and Teenage Childbearing." In *The Urban Underclass*, ed. Christopher Jencks and Paul Peterson. Washington, D.C.: Brookings Institution, 1991.

Crosbie, Paul V., and Dianne Bitte. "A Test of Luker's Theory of Contraceptive Risk-Taking." *Studies in Family Planning* 13, no. 3 (1982): 67–78.

Dalton, Harlon. "AIDS in Blackface." *Daedalus* 118, no. 3 (1989): 205–27.

Dash, Leon. *When Children Want Children.* New York: Morrow, 1989.

Davis, Angela Y. *Women, Culture, and Politics.* New York: Vintage Books, 1990.

Day, Randall D., and Wade C. Mackey. "Children as Resources: A Cultural Analysis." *Family Perspective* 20 (1988): 251–64.

De La Cancela, Victor. "Minority AIDS Prevention: Moving Beyond Cultural Perspectives towards Sociopolitical Empowerment." *AIDS Education and Prevention* 1, no. 2 (1989): 141–53.

De Lamater, John, and Patricia MacCorqodale. *Premarital Sexuality: Attitudes, Relationships, Behavior.* Madison: University of Wisconsin Press, 1979.

Des Jarlais, Don C., Samuel R. Friedman, and Cathy Casriel. "Target Groups for Preventing AIDS among Intravenous Drug Users: The 'Hard' Data Studies." *Journal of Consulting and Clinical Psychology* 58, no. 1 (1991): 50–56.

Des Jarlais, Don C., Susan Tross, and Samuel R. Friedman."Behavioral Change in Response to AIDS." In *AIDS and Other Manifestations of HIV Infection*, ed. G. P. Wormser, R. E. Stahl, and E. J. Battone. Park Ridge, N.J.: Noyes, 1987.

Diamond, Timothy, and Judith A. Levy. "Adulthood." In *Handbook of Behavioral Medicine in Women*, ed. E. A. Blechman and Kelly D. Brownell. New York: Pergamon, 1988.

DiClemente, Ralph J. "Predictors of HIV-Preventive Sexual Behavior in a High-Risk Adolescent Population: Influence of Perceived Peer Norms and Sexual Communication on Incarcerated Adolescents' Consistent Use of Condoms." *Society for Adolescent Medicine* 12 (1991): 385–90.

DiClemente, Ralph J., and G. M. Wingood. "A Randomized Controlled Trial of an HIV Sexual Risk-Reduction Intervention for Young African-American Women." *Journal of the American Medical Association* 274, no. 16 (1995): 1271–76.

Diorio, Joseph A. "Contraception, Copulation, Domination, and the Theoretical Barrenness of Sex Education Literature." *Educational Theory* 35, no. 3 (1985): 239–54.

Dore, Martha M., and Ana O. Dumois. "Cultural Differences in the Meaning of Adolescent Pregnancy." *Families in Society* (February 1990): 93–101.

Dryfoos, Joy G. *Adolescents at Risk: Prevalence and Prevention*. New York: Oxford University Press, 1990.

Duesberg, Peter H. "AIDS Epidemiology: Inconsistencies with Human Immunodeficiency Virus and with Infectious Disease." *National Academy of Science* 88 (1991): 1575–79.

Duneier, Mitchell. *Slim's Table: Race, Respectability, and Masculinity*. Chicago: University of Chicago, 1992.

Eakins, Pamela. *The American Way of Birth*. Philadelphia: Temple University Press, 1986.

Edelman, Marian Wright. "The Black Family in America." In *The Black Woman's Health Book*, ed. Evelyn White. Seattle: Seal, 1990.

Edelman, Peter, and Joyce Ladner. *Adolescence and Poverty: Challenge for the 1990's*. Washington, D.C.: Center for National Policy Press, 1991.

Eisen, Marvin, Gail L. Zellman, and Alfred L. McAlister. "Evaluating the Impact of a Theory-Based Sexuality and Contraceptive Education Program." *Family Planning Perspectives* 22, no. 6 (1990): 261–71.

Epstein, Steven. "Sexuality and Identity: The Contribution of Object Relations Theory to a Constructionist Sociology." *Theory and Society* 20 (1991): 825–73.

Facts on Working Women. *Black Women in the Labor Force*. Washington, D.C.: U.S. Department of Labor, 1991.

Fan, Hung, Ross F. Conner, and Luis P. Villarreal. *AIDS: Science and Society*. Sudbury, Mass.: Jones and Bertlet, 1998.

Feldman, Douglas. *Culture and AIDS*. New York: Praeger, 1990.

Fine, Michelle. "Sexuality, Schooling and Adolescent Females: The Missing Discourse of Desire." *Harvard Educational Review* 58, no. 1 (1988): 29–53.

Flaskerud, Jacquelyn H., and Adeline M. Nyamathi. "Black and Latina Women's AIDS Related Knowledge, Attitudes, and Practices." *Research in Nursing and Health* 12 (1989): 339–46.

Fleishman, John A. "Personality Characteristics and Coping Patterns." *Journal of Health and Social Behavior* 25 (1984): 229–44.

Ford, Kathleen, and Anne Norris. "Urban African-American and Hispanic Adolescents and Young Adults: Who Do They Talk to about AIDS and Condoms? What Are They Learning?" *AIDS Education and Prevention* 3, no. 2 (1991): 197–206.

Forste, Renata T., and Tim B. Heaton. "Initiation of Sexual Activity among Female Adolescents." *Youth and Society* 19, no. 3 (1988): 250–68.

Forste, Renata T., and Marta Tienda. "Race and Ethnic Variation in the Schooling Consequences of Female Adolescent Sexual Activity." *Social Science Quarterly* 73, no. 1 (1992): 12–30.

Fox, Greer Litton. "The Family's Role in Adolescent Sexual Behavior." In *Teenage Pregnancy in a Family Context*, ed. T. Ooms. Philadelphia: Temple University Press, 1981.

Francis, David, and Jean Chin. "Counselling the HIV-Positive Woman Regarding Pregnancy." *Journal of the American Medical Association* 257 (1987): 3361.

Frymier, Jack. *Growing Up Is Risky Business and Schools Are Not to Blame*, Vols. I and II. Bloomington, Ind.: Phi Delta Kappa, 1992.

Funch, Donna, and James Marshall. "Self-Reliance as a Modifier of the Effects of Life, Stress and Social Support." *Journal of Psychosomatic Research* 28 (1984): 9–15.

Furstenberg, Frank F. "As the Pendulum Swings: Teenage Childbearing and Social Concern." *Family Relations* 40 (1991): 127–38.

———. "Teenage Childbearing and Cultural Rationality: A Thesis in Search of Evidence." *Family Relations* 41 (1992): 239–43.

Furstenberg, Frank, Jeanne Brooks-Gunn, and Lindsay Chase-Lansdale. "Teenaged Pregnancy and Childbearing." *American Psychologist* 44, no. 2 (1989): 313–20.

Furstenberg, Frank, Richard Lincoln, and F. Mencken, eds. *Teenage Sexuality, Pregnancy and Childbearing*. Philadelphia: University of Philadelphia Press, 1981.

Galea, Robert P., Benjamin F. Lewis, and Lori A. Baker, eds. *AIDS and IV Drug Abusers: Current Perspectives*. Owing Mills, Md.: Rynd Communications, 1987.

Gallois, Cynthia, Yoshihisa Kashima, Deborah Terry, Malcolm McCamish, Perri Timmins, and Anita Chauvin. "Safe and Unsafe Sexual Intentions and Behavior: The Effects of Norms and Attitudes." *Journal of Applied Social Psychology* 22, no. 19 (1992): 1521–45.

Gamson, William, and A. Modigliani, eds. *Conceptions of Social Life*. New York: Little, Brown, 1974.

Gans, Herbert. *The War against The Poor: The Underclass and Antipoverty Policy*. New York; BasicBooks, 1995.

Gasch, Helen, D. Michael Poulson, Robert E. Fullilove, and Mindy Thompson Fullilove. "Shaping AIDS Education and Prevention Programs for African-Americans amidst Community Decline." *Journal of Negro Education* 60 (1991): 185–96.

Geertz, Clifford. *Negara*. Princeton, N.J.: Princeton University Press, 1980.

Geronimus, Arline. "On Teenage Childbearing and Neonatal Mortality in the United States." *Population and Development Review* 13, no. 2 (1987): 245–79.

———. "Teenage Childbearing and Social and Reproductive Disadavantage: The Evolution of Complex Questions and the Demise of Simple Answers." *Family Relations* 40 (1991): 463–71.

———. "Teenage Childbearing and Social Disadvantage: Unprotected Discourse." *Family Relations* 41 (1992): 244–48.

Ginzberg, Eli, Howard S. Berliner, and Miriam Ostow. *Young People at Risk: Is Prevention Possible?* Boulder, Colo.: Westview, 1988.

Giordano, Peggy, Stephen Cernkovich, and Alfred DeMaris. "The Family and Peer Relations of Black Adolescents." *Journal of Marriage and the Family* 55 (1993): 277–87.

Gordon, Lewis R. *Bad Faith and Antiblack Racism*. Atlantic Highlands, N.J.: Humanities Press, 1995.

Gordon, Lewis, and Abdullah Shabazz. "Brothers Getting Busy." New Haven, Conn.: Pamphlet, 1991.

Gordon, Linda. *Woman's Body, Woman's Right*. London: Penguin, 1977.

Gordon, Sol, and Jane F. Gilgun. "Adolescent Sexuality." In *Handbook of Adolescent Psychology*, ed. Vincent Van Hasselt and Michael Herson. New York: Pergamon, 1987.

Grimes, David. "The CDC and Abortion of HIV-Positive Women." *Journal of the American Medical Association* 258 (1987): 1176.

Grmek, Mirko D. *History of AIDS: Emergence and Origin of a Modern Pandemic*. Princeton, N.J.: Princeton University Press, 1990.

Hall, Elaine J., and Myra M. Ferree. "Race Differences in Abortion Attitudes." *Public Opinion Quarterly* 50 (1986): 193–207.

Hardy, Janet B., Anne K. Duggan, Katya Masnyk, and Carol Pearson. "Fathers of Children Born to Young Urban Mothers." *Family Planning Perspectives* 21, no. 4 (1989): 159–63.

Hare, Bruce. "African-American Youth at Risk." In *Teenage Pregnancy: Developmental Strategies for the Twenty First Century*, ed. Dionne Jones and Stanley F. Battle. New Brunswick, N.J.: Transaction, 1991.

Harlow, Caroline Wolf. *Female Victims of Violent Crime*. Washington, D.C.: U.S. Department of Justice, 1991.

Harris, Naomi Ruth. *Teen Pregnancy: An Examination of Related Factors*. New Haven, Conn.: Yale Medical School, 1991.

Hayward, Mark D., William R. Grady, and John O. G. Billy. "The Influence of Socioeconomic Status on Adolescent Pregnancy." *Social Science Quarterly* 73, no. 4 (1992): 750–72.

Heath, Shirley Brice, and Milbrey W. McLaughlin, eds. *Identity and Inner City Youth: Beyond Ethnicity and Gender*. New York: Teachers College Press, 1993.

Hein, Karen. "Fighting AIDS in Adolescents." *Issue in Science Technology* (Spring 1991): 67–72.

Hernton, Calvin C. *Sex and Racism in America*. New York: Anchor Books, 1965/1992.

Herz, Elicia J., and Janet S. Reis. "Family Life Education for Young Inner-City Teens: Identifying Needs." *Journal of Youth and Adolescence* 16, no. 4 (1987): 361–76.

Hochschild, Arlie. *The Second Shift: Work, Parenting and the Revolution at Home.* New York: Viking, 1989.

Honey, Ellen. "AIDS and the Inner City: Critical Issues." *Social Casework* 69 (1988): 365–70.

hooks, bell. *Yearning: Race, Gender, and Cultural Politics.* Boston: South End Press, 1990.

Human Resource Management News. "Family Friendly—But Not to All Families." Chicago: Remy, 1994.

Ickovics, Jeannette R., and Judith Rodin. "Women and AIDS in the United States: Epidemiology, Natural History and Mediating Mechanisims." *Health Psychology* 11, no. 1 (1992): 1–16.

Institute of Medicine, National Academy of Sciences. *Confronting AIDS: Directions for Public Health, Health Care, and Research.* Washington, D.C.: National Academy Press, 1986.

Ireson, Carol J. "Adolescent Pregnancy and Sex Roles." *Sex Roles* 11, no. 3/4 (1984): 189–201.

Ishii-Kuntz, Masako, Les B. Whitbeck, and Ronald L. Simons. "AIDS and Perceived Change in Sexual Practice: An Analysis of a College Sample from California and Iowa." *Journal of Applied Social Science* 20, no. 16 (1990): 1301–21.

Jadack, Rosemary A., Janet S. Hyde, and Mary L. Keller. "Gender and Knowledge about HIV, Risky Sexual Behavior, and Safer Sex Practices." *Research in Nursing Health* 18, no. 4 (1995): 313–24.

Jaffe, Leslie R., Mavis Seehaus, Caudia Wagner, and Bonnie Leadbeater. "Anal Intercourse and Knowledge of Acquired Immune Deficiency Syndrome among Minority-Group Female Adolescents." *Journal of Pediatrics* 112, no. 6 (1988): 1005–7.

Jaynes, Gerald D., and Robin Williams, Jr. *A Common Destiny: Blacks and American Society.* Washington, D.C.: National Academy Press, 1989.

Jeffery, Robert W. "Risk Behaviors and Health: Contrasting Individual and Population Perspectives." *American Psychologist* 44, no. 9 (1989): 1194–202.

Jencks, Christopher, and Paul E. Peterson. *The Urban Underclass.* Washington, D.C.: Brookings Institution, 1991.

Jewell, K. Sue. *Survival of the Black Family.* New York: Praeger, 1988.

———. *From Mammy to Miss America and Beyond: Cultural Images and the Shaping of U.S. Social Policy.* New York: Routlege, 1993.

Johnson, Ernest H., Larry Gant, Yvonne Hinkle, Douglas Gilbert, Cassandra Willis, and Tanya Hoopwood. "Do African-American Men and Women Differ in Their Knowledge about AIDS, Attitudes about Condoms, and Sexual Behaviors?" *Journal of the National Medical Association* 84, no. 1 (1992): 49–64.

Jones, Elise F., Jacqueline D. Forrest, Noreen Goldman, Stanley Henshaw, Richard Lincoln, Jeannie Rosoff, Charles Westoff, and Dierdre Wulf. *Teenage Pregnancy in Industrialized Countries.* New Haven, Conn.: Yale University Press, 1986.

Jorgensen, Stephen R. "Sex Education and the Reduction of Adolescent Pregnancies: Prospects for the 1980's." *Journal of Early Adolescence* 1, no. 1 (1981): 38–52.

Joseph, Jill G., Maurice Adib, James Koopman, and David Ostrow. "Behavior Change in Longitudinal Studies: Adoption of Condom Use by Homosexual/Bisexual Men." *American Journal of Public Health* 80, no. 12 (1990): 1513–14.

Joseph, Jill G., Carol Ann Emmons, Ronald Kessler, Camille B. Wortman, Keith O'Brien, William T. Hocker, and Catherine Schaefer. "Coping with the Threat of AIDS: An Approach to Psychosocial Assessment." *American Psychologist* 39 (1984): 11–21.

Jurich, Joan A., Rebecca A. Adams, and John E. Schulenberg. "Factors Related to Behavior Change in Response to AIDS." *Family Relations* 41 (1992): 97–103.

Kalmuss, Debra, Amelia I. Lawton, and Pearila Brickner Namerow. "Advantages and Disadvantages of Pregnancy and Contraception: Teenagers' Perceptions." *Population and Environment* 9, no. 1 (1987): 23–40.

Kantrowitz, Barbara. "Breaking the Poverty Cycle." *Newsweek* (May 28, 1990): 65.

Kaplan, Abraham. *The Conduct of Inquiry.* San Francisco: Chandler, 1964.

Kaplan, Edward H., and Paul Abramson. "So What If the Program Ain't Perfect? A Mathematical Model of AIDS Education." *Evaluation Review* 13, no. 2 (1989): 107–22.

Kaplan, Howard B., Carol A. Bailey, and William Simon. "The Sociological Study of AIDS: A Critical Review of the Literature and Suggested Research Agenda." *Journal of Health and Social Behavior* 28 (1987): 140–57.

Kaplan, Robert. "Behavior as the Central Outcome in Health Care." *American Psychologist* 45, no. 11 (1990): 1211–20.

Keller, Steven E., Jacqueline Bertlett, Steven J. Schleifer, Robert L. Johnson, Elizabeth Pinner, and Beverly Delaney. "HIV Relevant Sexual Behavior among a Healthy Inner-City Heterosexual Adolescent Population in an Endemic Area of HIV." *Journal of Adolescent Health* 12 (1991): 44–48.

Kelly, Jeffrey A., Janet St. Lawrence, Yolanda E. Diaz, L. Yvonne Stevenson, Allan C. Hauth, Ted L. Brasfield, Seth C. Kalichman, Joseph E. Smith, and Michael E. Andrews. "HIV Risk Behavior Reduction Following Interviews with Key Opinion Leaders of the Population: An Experimental Analysis." *American Journal of Public Health* 81, no. 2 (1991): 168–71.

Kirby, Douglas, Cynthia Waszak, and Julie Ziegler. "Six School-Based Clinics: Their Reproductive Health Services and Impact on Sexual Behavior." *Family Planning Perspectives* 23, no. 1 (1991): 6–16.

Klein, Hugh. "Adolescence, Youth and Young Adulthood: Rethinking Current Conceptualizations of Life Stage." *Youth and Society* 21, no. 4 (1990): 446–71.

Kotlowitz, Alex. *There Are No Children Here.* New York: Doubleday, 1991.

Koyle, Priscilla, Fay Carter, Larry C. Jensen, Joe Olsen, and Bert Cundick. "Comparison of Sexual Behaviors among Adolescents Having an Early, Middle and Late First Intercourse Experience." *Youth and Society* 20, no. 4 (1989): 461–76.

Ladner, Joyce A. "Black Teenage Pregnancy: A Challenge for Educators." *Journal of Negro Education* 56, no. 1 (1987): 53–63.

———. *Tomorrow's Tomorrow*. New York: Doubleday, 1995.

Landesman, Sheldon, A. Willoughby, and H. Minkoff. "HIV Disease in Reproductive Age Women: A Problem of the Present." *Journal of the American Medical Association* 261 (1989): 1326–27.

Lasker, Judith, and Susan Borg. *In Search of Parenthood*. Boston: Beacon, 1987.

Law, Ron. "Public Policy and Health Care Delivery: A Practitioner's Perspective." In *Slipping through the Cracks: The Status of Black Women*, ed. Margaret C. Simms and Julianne Malveaux. New Brunswick, N.J.: Transaction, 1986.

Leadbeater, Bonnie J. Ross, and Niobe Way, eds. *Urban Girls: Resisting Stereotypes, Creating Identities*. New York: New York University Press, 1996.

Leadership, Education, and Athletics in Partnership (LEAP). http://www.leap.yale.edu, Summer 1997.

Levine, Carol. "AIDS and Changing Concepts of Family." *Milbank Quarterly* 68 Suppl., no. 1 (1990): 33–57.

Levine, Sol, and James Sorenson. "Social and Cultural Factors in Health Promotion." In *Behavioral Health: A Handbook of Health Enhancement and Disease Prevention*, ed. J. D. Matarazzo, S. M. Weiss, J. A. Herd, N. E. Miller. New York: Wiley, 1984.

Lewis, Oscar. *Five Families: Mexican Case Study in the Culture of Poverty*. New York: Basic Books, 1959.

Liburd, Leandris C., and Janice V. Bowie. "Intentional Teenage Pregnancy: A Community Diagnosis and Action Plan." *Health Education* 20, no. 5 (1989): 33–38.

Lindsey, Linda. *Gender Roles: A Sociological Perspective*, 3rd edition. Upper Saddle River, N.J.: Prentice Hall, 1997.

Lloyd, Gary A. "HIV-Infection, AIDS and Family Disruption" In *The Global Impact of AIDS*, ed. A. F. Fleming. New York: Liss, 1988.

Lockett, Gloria. "Black Prostitutes and AIDS." In *The Black Woman's Health Book*, ed. Evelyn White. Seattle: Seal, 1990.

Loutrel, William F. *Directory of AIDS/HIV Resources and Services—South Central Connecticut*. Hartford: Infoline/United Way of Connecticut, 1991.

Lowenstein, George, and Frank Furstenberg. "Is Teenage Sexual Behavior Rational?" *Journal of Applied Social Psychology* 21, no. 12 (1991): 957–86.

Luker, Kristin. *Dubious Conceptions: The Politics of Teenage Pregnancy*. Cambridge, Mass.: Harvard University Press, 1997.

———. *Taking Chances: Abortion and the Decision Not to Contracept*. Berkeley: University of California Press, 1975.

Macklin, Eleanor D. "AIDS: Implication for Families." *Family Relations* 37 (1988): 141–49.

Mangano, Joseph J. "Young Adults in the 1980's: Why Mortality Rates Are Rising." *Health/PAC Bulletin* (Summer 1991): 19–24.

Mann, Jonathan, and Daniel Tarantola, eds. *AIDS in the World II: Global Dimensions, Social Roots, and Responses*. New York: Oxford University Press, 1996.

Marte, Carola, and Kathryn Anastos. "Women—The Missing Persons in the AIDS Epidemic (Part II)." *Health/Pac Bulletin* (Spring 1990): 11–18.

———. "Women—The Missing Persons in the AIDS Epidemic." *Health/Pac Bulletin* (Winter 1989): 6–13.

Maticka-Tyndale, Eleanor. "Modification of Sexual Activities in the Era of AIDS—A Trend Analysis of Adolescent Sexual Activity." *Youth and Society* 23, no. 1 (1991): 31–49.

Matzen, J. L. "Assessment of Human Immunodeficiency Virus/Acquired Immunodeficiency Syndrome Audiovisual Materials Designed for Grades 7 through 12." *Journal of Pediatric Nursing* 10, no. 2 (1995): 114–20.

Mayfield, Lorraine P. "Early Parenthood among Low Income Girls." In *The Black Family*, ed. Robert Staples. Belmont, Calif.: Wadsworth, 1986.

Mays, Vickie M., and Susan C. Cochran. "Issues in the Perception of AIDS Risk and Risk Reduction Activities by Black and Hispanic/Latina Women." *American Psychologist* 43 (1988): 949–57.

McAdoo, Harriet P. "Black Mothers and the Extended Family Support Network." In *The Black Woman*, ed. LaFrances Rogers-Rose. Beverly Hills: Sage, 1978.

McGinnis, J. M. "Health Objectives for the Nation." *American Psychologist* 46, no. 5 (1991): 520–24.

McKenry, Patrick. "Research on Black Adolescents: A Legacy of Cultural Bias." *Journal of Adolescent Research* 4 (1989): 254–64.

McKinney, Kathleen, and Susan Sprecher. "The Effect of Current Sexual Behavior on Friendship, Dating and Marriage Desirability." *Journal of Sex Research* 28 (1991): 387–408.

McLoyd, Vonnie, and Debra M. Hernandez Jozefowicz, "Sizing Up Their Future: Predictors of African American Adolescent Females' Expectancies about Their Economic Fortunes and Family Life Courses." In *Urban Girls: Resisting Stereotypes, Creating Identities*, ed. Bonnie J. Ross Leadbeater and Niobe Way. New York: New York University Press, 1996.

Miller, Brent C., and Kristin Moore. "Adolescent Sexual Behavior, Pregnancy and Parenting: Research through the 1980's." *Journal of Marriage and the Family* 52 (1990): 1025–44.

Miller, Brent C., Roger B. Christensen, and Terrance O. Olson. "Adolescent Self-Esteem in Relation to Sexual Attitudes and Behavior." *Youth and Society* 19, no. 1 (1987): 93–111.

Miller, Heather G., Charles F. Turner, and Lincoln E. Moses, eds. *AIDS in the Second Decade*. Washington, D.C.: National Academy Press, 1990.

Mitchell, Angela. "AIDS: We Are Not Immune." *Emerge* 2 (1990): 30–44.

Mitchell, Janet L. "Women, AIDS and Public Policy." *AIDS and Public Policy Journal* 3 (1988): 50–52.

Moore, Susan, and Doreen Rosenthal. *Sexuality in Adolescence*. New York: Routledge, 1993.

Morbidity and Mortality Weekly Report 46, no. 8. mmwr-asc@listserv.cdc.gov, February 28, 1997.

Morbidity and Mortality Weekly Report 45, September 27, 1996.

Morbidity and Mortality Weekly Report 45, no. 6, February 16, 1996.

Morbidity and Mortality Weekly Report 44, no. 2, May 5, 1995.

Morgan, W. Meade, and James W. Curran. "Acquired Immunodeficiency Syndrome: Current and Future Trends." *Public Health Reports* 101 (1986): 459–65.

Mosher, William D., and James W. McNally. "Contraceptive Use at First Premarital Intercourse: United States, 1965–1988." *Family Planning Perspectives* 23, no. 3 (1991): 108–116.

Moynihan, Daniel Patrick. *The Negro Family: The Case for National Action.* Washington, D.C.: Office of Policy Planning and Research, U.S. Department of Labor, 1965.

Moyse-Steinberg, Dominique. "A Model for Adolescent Pregnancy Prevention through the Use of Small Groups." *Social Work with Groups* 13, no. 2 (1990): 57–68.

Mullings, Leith. "Inequality and African-American Health Status: Policies and Prospects." In *Race: Twentieth Century Dilemma—Twenty First Century Prognoses*, ed. William Van Horne. Madison: University of Wisconsin Institute on Race and Ethnicity, 1989.

Murray, Charles. *Losing Ground: American Social Policy 1950–1980.* New York: Basic Books, 1995.

Murry, Velma McBride. "Incidence of First Pregnancy among Black Adolescent Females over Three Decades." *Youth and Society* 23, no. 4 (1992): 478–506.

Musick, Judith S. *Young, Poor and Pregnant: The Psychology of Teenage Motherhood.* New Haven, Conn.: Yale University Press, 1993.

Namerow, Pearila Brickner, Amelia Lawton, and Susan G. Philliber. "Teenagers' Perceived and Actual Probabilities of Pregnancy." *Adolescence* 22, no. 86 (1987): 475–85.

Nathanson, Constance. *Dangerous Passage: The Social Control of Sexuality in Women's Adolescence.* Philadelphia: Temple University Press, 1991.

National Center for Health Statistics—Advance Data. *AIDS Knowledge and Attitudes for January–March 1990.* Hyattsville, Md.: U.S. Department of Health and Human Services, 1990.

National Council of Negro Women. *Women of Color Reproductive Health Poll.* Washington, D.C.: National Council of Negro Women, 1991.

National Institutes of Health, Office of AIDS Research. "HIV/AIDS-Related Research Programs at the NIH." http//:www.os.dnhs.gov/, October 4, 1996.

Neighbors, Harold, and James Jackson. "The Use of Informal and Formal Help: Four Patterns of Illness Behavior in the Black Community." *American Journal of Community Psychology* 12 (1984): 629–44.

New Haven Census. "Income and Poverty Status in 1989." New Haven, CPH-L-83, Table 3 http://www.statlab.stat.yale.edu/cityroom/NHOL.html/, 1990

New York State Department of Health. *Overview of HIV Infection and AIDS: Participant's Manual.* New York: AIDS Institute, 1991.

Norwood, Christopher. *Advice for Life: A Woman's Guide to AIDS Risk Prevention.* New York: Pantheon, 1987.

Oakes, Jeannie. *Keeping Track: How Schools Structure Inequality.* New Haven, Conn.: Yale University Press, 1985.

Oakley, Ann. *Woman Confined: Towards a Sociology of Childbirth.* Oxford: Robertson, 1980.

Office of National AIDS Policy. *Youth and HIV/AIDS: An American Agenda—A Report to the President.* Washington, D.C.: National AIDS Fund, 1996.

Ogbu, John. *The Next Generation: An Ethnography of Education in an Urban Neighborhood.* London: Macmillan, 1974.

O'Keefe, Elaine, Edward Kaplan, and Kaveh Khoshnood. *Preliminary Report: City of New Haven Needle Exchange Program.* New Haven, Conn.: Mayor's Task Force on AIDS, 1991.

Ormond, Cheryl, Mary Luszcz, Leon Mann, and Gery Beswick. "A Metacognitive Analysis of Decision Making in Adolescents." *Journal of Adolescence* 14 (1991): 275–91.

Ortiz, Carmen G., and Ena Vazquez Nuttal. "Adolescent Pregnancy: Effects of Family Support, Education, and Religion on the Decision to Carry or Terminate among Puerto Rican Teenagers." *Adolescence* 22, no. 8 (1987): 897–917.

Paget, Kathleen. "Adolescent Pregnancy: Implications for Prevention Strategies in Educational Settings." *School Psychology Review* 17, no. 4 (1988): 570–80.

Palmer, Susan J. "AIDS as a Metaphor." *Society* 26 (1989): 44–50.

Perrin, Noel. "Let's Pay Teenage Women Not to Get Pregnant." *Newsday* (August 2, 1990): 63.

Perrow, Charles, and Mauro Guillen. *The AIDS Disaster.* New Haven, Conn.: Yale University Press, 1990.

Petchesky, Rosalind P. "Reproductive Freedom: Beyond a Woman's Right to Choose." *Signs* 5 (1980): 661–85.

Peterson, Paul E. *The New Urban Reality.* Washington, D.C.: Brookings Institution, 1985.

Pittman, Karen J. "Reading and Writing as Risk Reduction: The School's Role in Preventing Teenage Pregnancies." In *Teenage Pregnancy: Developmental Strategies for Change in the Twenty First Century,* ed. Dionne Jones and Stanley Battle. New Brunswick, N.J.: Transaction, 1991.

Poland, Marilyn. "Ethical Issues in the Delivery of Quality Care to Pregnant Indigent Women." In *New Approaches to Human Reproduction,* ed. Linda M. Whiteford and Marilyn L. Poland. Boulder, Colo.: Westview, 1989.

Pollitt, Katha. "A New Assault on Feminism." *The Nation* (March 26, 1990): 409–18.

Postman, Neil. *The Disappearance of Childhood.* New York: Vintage Books, 1994.

Quadagno, Jill. *The Color of Welfare: How Racism Undermined the War on Poverty.* New York: Oxford University Press, 1994.

Ratzan, Scott C. *AIDS: Effective Communication for the 90's.* Washington, D.C.: Taylor Francis, 1993.

Rawitscher, L. A., R. Saitz, and L. S. Friedman. "Adolescents' Preferences Regarding Human Immunodeficiency Virus (HIV)–Related Physician Counseling and HIV Testing." *Pediatrics* 96 (1995): 52–58.

Redmond, Marcia A. "Attitudes of Adolescent Males toward Adolescent Pregnancy and Fatherhood." *Family Relations* 34 (1985): 337–42.

Richie, Beth. "AIDS: In Living Color." In *The Black Woman's Health Book*, ed. Evelyn White. Seattle: Seal, 1990.

Robbins, Cynthia, Howard B. Kaplan, and Steven S. Martin. "Antecedents of Pregnancy Among Unmarried Adolescents." *Journal of Marriage and the Family* 47 (1985): 567–83.

Rodin, Judith, and Jeanette Ickovics. "Women's Health—Review and Research Agenda as We Approach the 21st Century." *American Psychologist* 45, no. 9 (1990): 1018–34.

Rogers, M. "Controlling Perinatally Acquired HIV Infection." *Western Journal of Medicine* 147 (1987): 109–10.

Rosenberg, Morris, and Ralph Turner, eds. *Social Psychology: Sociological Perspectives*. New York: Basic Books, 1981.

Rosenheim, Margaret, and Mark F. Testa, eds. *Early Parenthood and Coming of Age in the 1990's*. New Brunswick, N.J.: Rutgers University Press, 1993.

Rothman, Robert A. *Inequality and Stratification in the United States*. Upper Saddle River, N.J.: Prentice Hall, 1988.

Sapiro, Virginia. *Women in American Society*. Palo Alto, Calif.: Mayfield Publishing Co., 1986.

Schechter, Martin T., E. Jeffries, P. Constance, B. Douglas, S. Fay, M. Maynard, R. Nitz, B. Willough, W. Boyko, and A. Macleod. "Changes in Sexual Behavior and Fear of AIDS." *Lancet* 1 (1984): 1293.

Schinke, Steven P., Gilbert Botvin, Mario A. Orlandi, Robert F. Schilling, and Adam N. Gordon. "African-American and Hispanic-American Adolescents, HIV Infection and Preventative Intervention." *AIDS Education and Prevention* 2, no. 4 (1990): 305–12.

Scott-Jones, Diane. "Adolescent Childbearing: Risk and Resilience." *Education and Urban Society* 24, no. 1 (1991): 53–64.

Scott-Jones, Diane, and Anne B. White. "Correlates of Sexual Activity in Early Adolescence." *Journal of Early Adolescence* 10, no. 2 (1990): 221–38.

Selwyn, Peter, Ellie E. Schoenbaum, Katherine D. Davenny, Vera J. Robertson, Anat R. Feingold, J. S. Schulman, M. M. Mayers, R. S. Klein, G. H. Friedland, and M. F. Rogers. "Prospective Study of Human Immunodeficiency Virus Infection and Pregnancy Outcomes in Intravenous Drug Users." *Journal of the American Medical Association* 261 (1989): 1289–94.

Shayne, Vivian T., and Barbara J. Kaplan. "AIDS Education for Adolescents." *Youth and Society* 20, no. 2 (1988): 180–208.

Shelp, Earl, Edwin DuBose, and Ronald H. Sunderland. "AIDS and the Church: A Status Report." *Christian Century* 107, no. 35 (1990): 1135–37.

Slonim-Nevo, Vered, Martha N. Ozawa, and Wendy F. Auslander. "Knowledge, Attitudes and Behavior Related to AIDS among Youth in Residential Centers: Results from an Explanatory Study." *Journal of Adolescence* 14 (1991): 17–33.

Solinger, Rickie. "Race and 'Value': Black and White Illegitimate Babies, 1945–1965." In *Mothering: Ideology, Experience and Agency*, ed. Evelyn Nagano Glenn, Grace Chang, and Linda Rennie Forcey. New York: Routledge, 1994.

Solomon, Mildred Z., and W. DeLong. "Recent Sexually Transmitted Disease

Prevention Efforts and Their Implications for AIDS Health Education."
Health Education Quarterly 13 (1986): 301–16.

Sonenstein, Freya L., Joseph Pleck, and Leighton C. Ku. "Sexual Activity, Condom Use and AIDS Awareness among Adolescent Males." *Family Planning Perspectives* 21, no. 4 (1989): 152–58.

Spallone, Patricia. *Beyond Conception: The New Politics of Reproduction.* Granby, Mass.: Bergin & Garvey, 1989.

Stack, Carol. *All Our Kin: Strategies for Survival in a Black Community.* New York: Harper & Row, 1974.

————. "Black Kindreds: Parenthood and Personal Kindreds Among Urban Blacks." *Journal of Comparative Family Studies* 3 (1972): 194–206.

Stack, Carol, and Linda M. Burton. "Kinscripts: Reflections on Family, Generation, and Culture." In *Mothering: Ideology, Experience, and Agency,* ed. Evelyn Nakano Glenn, Grace Chang, and Linda Rennie Forcey. New York: Routledge, 1994.

Stall, Ron, Maria Eckstrand, Lance Pollack, Leon McKusick, and Thomas J. Coates. "Relapse from Safer Sex: The Next Challenge for AIDS Prevention Efforts." *Journal of AIDS* 3 (1990): 1181–87.

Stanton, Bonita F., X. Li, Izabel Ricardo, Jennifer Galbraith, Susan Feigelman, and Linda Kaljee. "A Randomized, Controlled Effectiveness Trial of an AIDS Prevention Program for Low-Income African American Youths." *Archive of Pediatric Adolescent Medicine* 150, no. 4 (1996): 363–72.

Staples, Robert. *The Black Family: Essays and Studies.* Belmont, Calif.: Wadsworth, 1986.

Staples, Robert, and Leanor Boulin Johnson. *Black Families at the Crossroads: Challenges and Prospects.* San Francisco: Jossey-Bass, 1993.

State of Connecticut Department of Health Services—AIDS Division. *AIDS in Connecticut—Annual Surveillance Report.* Hartford, Conn.: Department of Health Services, 1993.

Stern, Marilyn, and Aracelly Alvarez. "Knowledge of Child Development and Caretaking Attitudes: A Comparison of Pregnant, Parenting, and Nonpregnant Adolescents." *Family Relations* 41 (1992): 297–302.

Stevenson, Howard C. "The Role of the African-American Church in Education about Teenage Pregnancy." *Counseling and Values* 34 (1990): 130–33.

Subcommittee on Public Assistance and Unemployment Compensation of the Committee on Ways and Means. "Teenage Pregnancy Issues Hearings." House of Representatives (May 7, 1985): 1–4, 21–69, 92–127, 213–28; Y4.W36: 99–33.

Sullivan, T. Richard. "The Challenge of HIV Prevention among High-Risk Adolescents." *Health and Social Work* 21, no. 1 (1996): 58–65.

Sunderland Alan, G. Moroso, M. Berthaud, S. Holman, F. Cancellieri, H. Mendez, S. Landesman, and H. Minkoff. "Influence of HIV Infection on Pregnancy Decisions." In *Fourth International Conference on AIDS Stockholm.* Abstract 6607. Stockholm: 1988.

Susser, Ida. "The Separation of Mothers and Children." In *The Dual City,* ed. Manuel Castells and T. Mollenkopf. Beverly Hills: Sage, 1991.

Sy, Francisco S., Donna L. Richter, and A. Gene Copello. "Innovative Educational Strategies and Recommendations for AIDS Prevention and Control." *AIDS Education and Prevention* 1, no. 1 (1989): 53–6.

Taylor, Robert J. "African-American Inner City Youth and Subculture." In *Teenage Pregnancy: Developmental Strategies for Change in the Twenty First Century*, ed. Dionne J. Jones and Stanley F. Battle. New Brunswick, N.J.: Transaction, 1991.

———. "Receipt of Support from Family among Black Americans: Demographic and Familial Differences." *Journal of Marriage and the Family* 48 (1986): 67–77.

Taylor, Robert J., Linda M. Chatters, and Vickie M. Mays. "Parents, Children, Siblings, In-Laws, and Non-Kin as Sources of Emergency Assistance to Black Americans." *Family Relations* 37 (1988): 298–304.

Taylor, Robert J., Linda M. Chatters, M. Belinda Tucker, and Edith Lewis. "Development in Research on Black Families." *Journal of Marriage and the Family* 52 (1990): 993–1014.

Taylor, Shelley. "Health Psychology, the Science and the Field." *American Psychologist* 45, no. 1 (1990): 40–50.

Temoshok, Lydia, and Andrew Baum, eds. *Psychosocial Perspectives on AIDS—Etiology, Prevention and Treatment*. Hillsdale, N.J.: Erlbaum, 1990.

Thompson, Sharon. *Going All the Way: Teenage Girls' Tales of Sex, Romance, and Pregnancy*. New York: Hill & Wang, 1995.

Tolman, Deborah. "Adolescent Girls' Sexuality: Debunking the Myth of the Urban." In *Urban Girls: Resisting Stereotypes, Creating Identities*, ed. Bonnie J. Ross Leadbeater and Niobe Way. New York: New York University Press, 1996.

Tuhus, Melinda. "Our Youth at Risk: Children, Sex and Death in the Age of AIDS." *New Times Connecticut* (November 28–December 5, 1991): 8–12, 14.

Ture, Kwame, and Charles V. Hamilton. *Black Power*. New York: Vintage Books, 1992.

Turner, Jonathan. *The Structure of Sociological Theory*. Homewood, Ill.: Dorsey, 1982.

Vance, Susan, R.N., M.P.H., State of Connecticut Department of Health, AIDS Epidemiology Program. Personal interview, March 9, 1998.

Wallace, Helen M., George M. Ryan, Jr., and Allan C. Ogelsby, eds. *Maternal and Child Health Practices*. Oakland, Calif.: Third Party, 1988.

Wallace, John M., and Jerald Bachman. "Explaining Racial/Ethnic Differences in Adolescent Drug Use: The Impact of Background and Lifestyle." *Social Problems* 38, no. 3 (1991): 333–57.

Wallace, Rodrick, and Deborah Wallace. "Contagious Urban Decay and the Collapse of Public Health." *Health/PAC Bulletin* (Summer 1991): 13–18.

Washington, Anita C. "A Cultural and Historical Perspective on Pregnancy-Related Activity among U.S. Teenagers." *The Journal of Black Psychology* 9, no. 1 (1982): 1–28.

Weeks, Margaret R., Jean Schensul, Sunyna S. Williams, Merrill Singer, and Maryland Grier. "AIDS Prevention for African-American and Latina

Women: Building Culturally and Gender-Appropriate Intervention." *AIDS Education and Prevention* 7, no. 3 (1995): 251–63.

Weiner, Roberta. *AIDS: Impact on the Schools.* Arlington, Va.: Education Research Group, 1986.

White, Renée T. "In the Name of Love and Survival: Interpretations of Sexual Violence among Young Black American Women." In *Spoils of War: Women of Color, Cultures and Revolutions,* ed. T. Denean Sharpley Whiting and Renée T. White. Lanham, Md.: Rowman & Littlefield, 1997.

———. "Talking about Sex and HIV: Conceptualizing a New Sociology of Experience." In *Oral Narrative Research with Black Women: Collecting Treasures,* ed. Kim Marie Vaz. Thousand Oaks, Calif.: Sage, 1997.

Whitten, Norman E., and John F. Szwed. *Afro-American Anthropology.* New York: Free Press, 1970.

Williams, Linda S. "AIDS Risk Reduction: A Community Health Education Intervention for Minority High Risk Group Members." *Health Education Quarterly* 13 (1986): 407–21.

Williams, Terry, and William Kornblum. *The Uptown Kids: Struggle and Hope in the Projects.* New York: Putnam, 1994.

Wilson, William Julius. *The Truly Disadvantaged.* Chicago: University of Chicago Press, 1987.

Winter, Laraine, and Lynne Cooper Brekenmaker. "Tailoring Family Planning Services to the Special Needs of Adolescents." *Family Planning Perspectives* 23, no. 1 (1991): 24–30.

Witwer, M. "Pregnancy Risk Lessened for Teenagers with High Educational Aspirations." *Family Planning Perspectives* 25, no. 4 (1993): 189–90.

W.O.R.L.D. Newsletter. September 1991.

Worth, Dooley, and Ruth Rodriguez. "Latina Women and AIDS." *Radical America* 20 (1987): 63–67.

Wulfert, Edelgard, and Choi K. Wan. "Safer Sex Intentions and Condom Use, Viewed from a Health Belief, Reasoned Action, and Social Cognitive Perspective." *Journal of Sex Research* 32, no. 4 (1995): 299–311.

Wyatt, Gail Elizabeth. "Examining Ethnicity v. Race in AIDS Related Research." *Social Science Medicine* 33, no. 1 (1991): 37–45.

Yow, Valerie Raleigh. *Recording Oral History: A Practical Guide for Social Scientists.* Thousand Oaks, Calif.: Sage, 1994.

Zabin, Laurie Schwab, and Marilyn B. Hirsch. *Evaluation of Pregnancy Prevention Programs in the School Context.* Lexington, Mass.: Lexington Books, 1988.

Zelizer, Viviana. *Pricing the Priceless Child.* New York: Basic Books, 1985.

Zelnik, Melvin, John F. Kantner, and Kathleen Ford. *Sex and Pregnancy in Adolescence.* Thousand Oaks, Calif.: Sage, 1981.

Index

About the Author

Renée T. White is assistant professor of sociology at Central Connecticut State University in New Britain, Conn. She is co-editor of *Fanon: A Critical Reader* and *Spoils of War: Women of Color, Cultures, and Revolutions* (Rowman & Littlefield).